new heal

Visions of primary care

Edited by Tom Coffey GP, Guy Boersma, Linda Smith & Peter Wallace

New Health Network
165a Mermaid Court
Borough High Street
London SE1H 1HH
Tel and fax: 020 750 48677
coordinator@newhealthnetwork.co.uk
www.newhealthnetwork.co.uk

Published on behalf of New Health Network by:
King's Fund Publishing
11-13 Cavendish Square
London W1M OAN

© New Health Network 1999

All rights reserved.

First published 1999

No part of this publication may be reproduced, stored in a retrieval system or transmitted, in any form or by any means, electronic or mechanical, photocopying, recording and/or otherwise without the prior written permission of New Health Network.

This book may not be lent, resold, hired out or otherwise disposed of, without the prior written consent of New Health Network.

ISBN 1 85717 408 9

A CIP catalogue record for this book is available from the British Library.
Printed and bound in Great Britain.

Contents

Acknowledgements	6
Foreword *by The Right Honourable Tony Blair MP*	7
Introduction	10

1 Improving quality, access and structure — 15
TOM COFFEY
GP & Chair, Balham, Tooting & Wandsworth PCG
Virtual PCG Board Chair

'The word "quality" is bandied about so frequently that it can lose its meaning. Quality in primary care will have tangibility.'

2 Co-operative working relationships — 20
MICHAEL DIXON
GP & Chair, NHS Alliance
Virtual PCG Board GP Member

'The "responsible patient view" will increasingly dominate the pattern of services ... patients will see themselves less as individual consumers ... and more as NHS citizens ...'

3 We need to guarantee uniform quality — 24
HOWARD FREEMAN
GP & Co-chair, Nelson PCG
Virtual PCG Board GP Member

'The future for primary care must be about delivering a service of uniform quality nationally but how that is achieved will depend very much on local circumstances.'

4 The impact of information technology on health care — 28
PAUL CUNDY
GP & Chair, IM&T subcommittee of BMA's General Practitioners Committee
Virtual PCG Board GP Member

'Clinical decision support systems such as those first brought to the UK by NHS Direct and the co-operative movement in the late 1990s soon found general acceptance among professionals and within a few years they were extended beyond diagnostic advice to treatment management.'

5 New models of primary care 32

DAVID COLIN-THOMÉ
GP & Director of Primary Care, NHS Executive London
Virtual PCG Board GP Member

> 'A new primary care beckons, encompassing the attributes of traditional general practice, varied but information-linked ... first contact points for patients, radically re-designed hospital care funded by primary care trusts and a public health focus that links health care to the wider health agenda.'

6 Shifting professional roles in the primary health care team 36

TOBY LIPMAN
GP & Research Training Fellow, NHS Executive Northern & Yorkshire
Virtual PCG Board GP Member

> 'The time has come for a shifting of roles in primary care, and the removal of GPs from their central position ... Primary care groups ... will employ a range of professionals ... and must develop means of identifying who can most benefit each patient.'

7 The best care within finite resources 40

GILL FRASER
GP & Medical Director, Northumbria Healthcare NHS Trust
Virtual PCG Board GP Member

> 'Traditional primary and secondary care boundaries will disappear ... Joint training and rotation of posts through primary, community and secondary care will be necessary to develop common understanding and maintain standards.'

8 Patient-centred care – a new paradigm 43

BRIAN FISHER
GP & Vice Chair, South Lewisham PCG
Virtual PCG Board GP Member

> 'Accountability, sharing decision-making and planning result in professionals relinquishing control in favour of lay people.'

9 NICE's role in unlocking potential 47

ANDREW DILLON
Chief Executive, National Institute for Clinical Excellence (NICE)
Virtual PCG Board Chief Executive

> 'Remote access to specialists will speed diagnosis and treatment guidelines will allow more care to be provided from primary care medical centres.'

10 A perspective from a community trust 50

LUCY HADFIELD
Chief Executive, South West London Community NHS Trust
Virtual PCG Board Community Trust Member

> 'If the benefits of service changes are not clearly understood, health buildings disproportionately symbolise the NHS in the minds of the public and local politicians and any change is fiercely resisted. We need innovation and investment across all health care players to make the changes to buildings we need and to carry the public with us.'

11 Radical and imaginative initiatives 55

LYNN YOUNG

Community Health Advisor, Royal College of Nursing
Virtual PCG Board Nurse Member

> 'Well informed optimists working in the NHS believe that the current health and social policies are right and that primary health care workers have a new and huge opportunity to help improve the nation's health.'

12 Nurse-led primary care 59

SUE BAKER

Health Visitor, South West London Community NHS Trust
Virtual PCG Board Nurse Member

> 'Primary care groups have ... created new opportunities for nurses and will have a profound effect on the way primary care is provided by 2009 ... with an opportunity to extend their roles in the leadership and strategic development of primary care services.'

13 The ideal primary care service 61

DONNA COVEY

Director, Association of Community Health Councils of England & Wales
Virtual PCG Board Lay Member

> 'In my 2009, patients are the experts. Not just in the needs of our own condition, but in the strategic needs of our own communities as well.'

14 Lambeth in 2009 65

JUDITH BRODIE

Secretary for Social Services and Health Improvement, London Borough of Lambeth
Virtual PCG Board Social Services Member

> 'Technology has transformed the way we do things ... users and the public can regularly be consulted about borough or neighbourhood priorities.'

15 Community pharmacy 2009: would you believe it? 68

COLIN BALDWIN

Pharmacy Development Controller, Boots
Virtual PCG Board co-opted Community Pharmacist

> '... it was the creation of primary care groups and the re-engineering of primary and social care that provided the opportunity for community pharmacists to become partners in the planning and delivery of health care for the community.'

acknowledgements

Thanks to the corporate supporters of New Health Network, whose support has made this publication possible: Access Health UK, Boots, BSA, British Telecom, KPMG, Nabarro Nathanson, Quest, Superdrug.

Recognition is also due to the New Health Network Executive, whose efforts have made this publication possible: Hugh Blair, Dr Tom Coffey, Brian Flood, Lord Toby Harris, Professor David Kerr, Jo Lenaghan, Dr Chai Patel CBE, Claire Perry and Linda Smith.

<<< foreword >>>

Family doctors and nurses have been the backbone of the NHS since it was founded. Every day over 1 million people either visit their local surgery or receive a visit from their local doctor or nurse. Surveys consistently show that the public places a high level of trust in their GP.

The British primary care system has very many strengths and is admired throughout the world, and we need to hold on to all that is good about our current arrangements. For example, I see the continuity of care provided by the list system remaining at the heart of primary health care.

But the world is changing. Primary care services need to modernise if they are to maintain the same level of public support for the next 50 years as they have done for the last 50. That is why I welcome this book as it looks ahead at what might happen over the next decade. I hope that it will spark a debate about the future direction of family health services.

I know that some will say the problem is that we have too much change and that the best thing the politicians could do would be to leave doctors to get on and care for their patients. But that would be to run away from the challenges that we face. It would also fail to serve the interests of patients.

Change is taking place on many fronts. People's lifestyles are changing. Many more women now go out to work than 20 years ago. That by itself has enormous implications for how we provide health care for those women and their children. In addition, the advent of Sunday shopping, 24-hour telephone banking and extended opening hours mean that people expect services in the public sector to be as accessible as in the private sector. The Internet, digital TV and telemedicine are opening up new ways to deliver health care and keep health professionals better informed about good medical practice. And the public is now much more demanding of the quality it expects, not just from doctors and nurses but from all professionals.

Many practices are rising to the challenge of modernisation. They have developed new clinics and services to meet their patients' needs. They have used the personal medical services scheme to develop hundreds of new ways of providing primary care to those who tend to get overlooked by the existing system. Flexible team working between GPs and practice and community nurses, physiotherapists and other health staff is now commonplace. Local GPs and nurses are at the forefront of making such a success of NHS Direct and introducing walk-in centres. And increasingly we are seeing hospital and family doctors getting together to cut waiting times and improve the way their patients receive diagnosis and care.

Modernising 1000 GP surgeries, providing a desktop computer for every GP and employing 500 extra practice nurses – which we are committed to doing over the next three years – will all help this process of change.

Primary care groups provide just the right vehicle for family doctors and their teams to build on all this good work. Already PCGs are bringing together the best of what is happening in each locality and making sure that everyone in an area can benefit from it. They are also putting doctors and nurses in the driving seat in shaping the way health care is organised to meet local needs. They will be able to use their financial control, coupled with information on costs and quality, to make sure their patients get efficient, convenient and quality hospital treatment.

PCGs will also bring a more systematic and clinically rigorous approach to managing chronic diseases like heart disease and diabetes. By using the best evidence-based medical standards and by working with hospitals, specialist centres and community teams, they will ensure that the different parts of the health care system – from self-care to advanced surgical procedures – work together to deliver a package of care designed to meet a patient's individual needs.

And as PCGs progress to primary care trusts there will be further opportunities to improve the way primary care works with community health services and social services.

Where might all this lead over the next ten years? People as a matter of routine will get instant access to health care advice over the phone through NHS Direct or through the Internet using NHS Direct On Line. When they need urgent treatment NHS Direct will, in partnership with GPs, arrange this as well. The important point about these services is that, as well as making the health service more convenient and accessible, they will also steer patients towards the most appropriate point in the health care system for them to use.

A combination of walk-in centres and more flexible opening times for surgeries will make it easier for people to fit health care needs into their busy lives. Nurses will take on more of the routine and minor ailment workload, with doctors spending more time with those patients whose symptoms require a GP's unique blend of knowledge and expertise. Electronic patient records will enable GPs to maintain continuity of care and knowledge of their patients even though their patients may be contacting the NHS through a more diverse set of services.

There will be more one-stop centres with doctors, dentists, pharmacists, opticians and other health services all on the one site, providing easy access to a range of health care.

Every GP will have a desktop PC linked to NHS Net to help with diagnosing and prescribing. And the technology will mean that the consulting room will be the place where appointments for outpatients and operations are booked, test results received and more diagnosis carried out using video and telelinks to hospital specialists.

Patients will have the assurance of knowing that their doctor and surgery are providing quality care, as all practices work to clear and recognised standards and GPs, like all doctors, have to demonstrate to their professional body every five years that they are fit to practise.

In most places the practice team will work on an integrated basis with community nurses, physiotherapists and social care staff to provide a wider range of preventive and rehabilitation services to elderly people in their own homes and in supported accommodation. People with chronic conditions such as diabetes, asthma, depression and heart disease will have much more regular help from the local health team in maintaining as healthy and full a lifestyle as possible. There will also be close links with schools, big employers and local councils to help promote healthy living and tackle some of the underlying causes of ill health.

General practice will continue to offer a variety of ways of working. Independent contractors, locally based contracts – like those in the personal medical services pilots – and salaried doctors will deliver services in a way that fits the needs of both patients and doctors.

This book sets out lots of interesting and exciting ideas. I want local GPs, nurses and primary care groups to join in the debate; not to be frightened or daunted by the challenge of the future, but to take the lead in shaping it.

Tony Blair

The Right Honourable Tony Blair MP

‹‹‹ Introduction ›››

'What do we mean by primary care? Primary or essential health care is the first level of contact of individuals, the family and community with the health system, bringing health care as close as possible to where people live and work; it is the first evidence of a continuing health care process. It needs participation at a local level in the planning and implementation of change, to provide services such as clean water, good food, education and sanitation.'

Source: World Health Organisation. *Report of International Conference on Primary Medical Care.* Geneva, 1978.

At the 60th anniversary of the NHS in 2008, we want to see a National Health Service that is once again the most respected organisation in the UK, and the nation's proudest asset. We are confident that this can be achieved, but only if it responds to the modernisation challenge. Primary care is at the heart of our health service. If the NHS is to modernise to meet the needs of patients in the 21st century, then primary care must be at the forefront of change.

Primary care is already leading the modernisation agenda through innovative developments such as NHS Direct, Booked Admissions projects and local primary care group initiatives. But this is merely the tip of the iceberg – there is much more to be done.

New Health Network (NHN) is publishing this collection of *Visions of Primary Care* to stimulate the debate and provide a space for thinking that will be necessary to achieve genuine change in the health service. We invited health care practitioners and patients to tell us their visions for primary care. Our aim was to create a 'virtual' Primary Care Group Board, representing the wide range of perspectives and views that will shape the development of primary care in the next century. We have not selected or edited according to political or professional views. Our criteria for inclusion has been that the submissions are thought provoking and forward looking. The result is a fascinating collection of views and visions on the future of primary care, not from policy analysts or politicians, but from the real experts: the professionals who provide care and the patients who access it.

In predicting the future, the writers range from those who anticipate that GPs will continue to have a central role, to those who anticipate nurse-led primary care. Others suggest that patients will be the experts of the future, and predict the development of Patient-centred primary care. Some contributors even anticipate the development of 'virtual primary care', with boundaries between primary and secondary care disappearing. A number of themes recur throughout this collection of visions, anticipating:

> more user-friendly primary care

> more integrated care, designed around the needs and circumstances of individual users

> easier access to care, resulting particularly from enhancements in information technology

> an increase in the range of health care services that will be provided by primary care practitioners and in primary care settings

> an increasingly multidisciplinary primary care workforce in 2009

> nurses with extended skills, responsibilities and training

> the continuation of the 'gatekeeping' responsibilities of primary care

> greater integration between health and social services planning and provision.

There are also a number of tensions that recur within some of the visions. We anticipate these to be key areas of debate in the next decade. These tensions include:

> the pursuit of uniformly high quality primary care in a manner which does not impede local flexibility and innovation

> the potential loss of 'the personal touch' as some primary care is provided via telephone helplines and information technology, to offer the benefits of more convenient and faster access to primary care advice and information

> the fact that the potential for primary care to deliver an expanded range of health care services will only become a reality if there is sufficient capacity in primary care to fulfil this potential.

Although the views published here are wide-ranging and diverse, the contributors all share a genuine optimism about the future and a belief in the ability of the NHS to modernise to meet the needs of patients in the 21st century.

All views published here are of course those of the authors alone and New Health Network is delighted to publish them in the spirit of debate. There is no one right answer; all are authentic voices and the personal views of primary care stakeholders representing a virtual PCG Board looking to the future.

We hope you will find the collected visions a stimulating read. We encourage you to participate in the discussion that these visions will provoke and to continue working with others to make the vision of modernisation a reality.

What is New Health Network?

The Network is a broad coalition of individuals and corporate supporters strongly committed to modernising the NHS. It is an inclusive alliance of the public, clinicians, NHS staff, unions and industry. The Executive Group is chaired by Claire Perry, Chief Executive of Bromley Health Authority. Our primary care champions include Dr Tom Coffey GP and Linda Smith, Chair of Lambeth, Southwark & Lewisham Health Authority. They are the inspirations behind this book and the Primary Care Listening Event, at which the publication was launched. The Executive is advised by a Reference Group comprising:

Mr Hugh Blair	*Partner, KPMG*
Mr Paul Castle	*Castle Communications*
Mr Geoffrey Filkin	*New Local Government Network*
Mr Brian Flood	*Chair, Northumbria Healthcare NHS Trust*
Lord Toby Harris	*House of Lords*
Professor David Kerr	*CRC Institute for Cancer Studies, University Of Birmingham*
Dr Tom Coffey	*Chair, Balham, Tooting & Wandsworth Primary Care Group*
Ms Jo Lenaghan	*Research Fellow, Institute for Public Policy Research*
Ms Sue Page	*Chief Executive, Northumbria Healthcare NHS Trust*
Mr Greg Parston	*Public Management Foundation*
Dr Chai Patel CBE	*Chief Executive, Westminster Health Care*
Ms Claire Perry	*Chief Executive, Bromley Health Authority*
Dr Peter Reading	*Chief Executive, University College London Hospitals NHS Trust*
Ms Linda Smith	*Chair, Lambeth, Southwark & Lewisham Health Authority*

Guy Boersma and Peter Wallace are the Network Co-ordination Team. Guy joined KPMG's Government Consulting team from the NHS, where he was Head of Commissioning at Worcester & District Authority. Peter is also a member of KPMG's Government Consulting team. He has undertaken a number of consultancy assignments for the Department of Health.

New Health Network is *independent.* Our aims have support across the political spectrum.

What are our aims?

New Health Network exists to encourage the NHS to fulfil its potential by stimulating an environment of innovation and change in the NHS for the benefit of patients. The Network acts, through conferences and publications such as this, as a facilitator and playmaker:

- creating a mechanism for open debate and thinking time at the grassroots
- challenging, educating and speculating on key issues
- championing change
- engendering debate and understanding of the big picture
- inspiring belief, confidence and enthusiasm in what is possible
- highlighting and spreading innovative practice.

How do I get involved?

If you support our aims and want to get involved, join our mailing list and participate in future New Health Network events.

To participate in the debate on the future of primary care, submit a response or a vision to us and the Network will distribute your views on our web site.

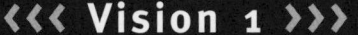

Improving quality, access and structure

Tom Coffey
GP & Chair, Balham, Tooting & Wandsworth PCG
Virtual PCG Board Chair

PRIMARY HEALTH CARE IS UNDERGOING A QUIET REVOLUTION. THE STATE OF FLUX IS UNSETTLING many practitioners and making them cling to their past. However, we know that primary care needs to change and modernise. We need to resolve this dichotomy by producing a vision for primary care that we can aspire to.

Most institutions are struggling to keep up with a rapidly changing society. Primary care is no exception. The public work long hours, change jobs and move frequently. **We expect responsive consumer friendly services, use IT on a daily basis and expect the best. Primary care will need to adapt to ensure it offers the services people need.**

I believe that the three key areas for primary care over the next decade will be improving quality, access and structure. The primary care of the future needs to have quality at its core. Access into primary care, and if necessary secondary care, will need to be extended to ensure all users of health care can get to see a doctor or nurse. There will not be a standard way of delivering care but we will expect care of a certain standard. The structure of primary care will evolve to allow changes to happen more easily. The gatekeeper role will remain pivotal and integration of all services will thus be crucial.

Quality

The word 'quality' is bandied around so frequently that it can lose its meaning. Quality in primary care will have tangibility. Practices are likely to have annual clinical governance agreements. They will encompass:

- implementation of NICE guidelines

- adherence to National Service Frameworks

- action plans in response to the recent Commission for Health Improvement visit

- re-accreditation plans for all health professionals

- implementation of the Health Improvement Programme (HImP) action plan

- locally agreed quality initiatives

The Royal College of General Practitioners has developed a practice accreditation scheme that identifies quality in services in general practice. Practices will use this model to ensure high standards. Each practice will have a professional personally accountable for quality. A practice based incentive scheme will be in place to promote modernisation.

Access

One of our greatest challenges is to improve access without undermining the basic tenets of general practice – continuity of care and effective gatekeeping. Poor access to primary care is one of the greatest causes of health inequality. Uptake of primary care is low among refugees, the homeless, the mentally ill, and adolescents. The challenge to increase access for primary care is not just to please the high-flying executive but to improve the health of the most underprivileged in society.

Improvement in access may be divided into 'practice based' and 'practice linked'.

Practice based changes may see extension of opening times, accessible translation services and flexible appointment systems. The primary care trust (PCT) may wish to co-ordinate a rota system of late and early opening. Secure connections between practices will allow sharing of patient information and continuity of care.

Practice linked improved access will be based around NHS Direct and walk-in clinics. These offer enormous potential. NHS Direct will work in partnership with the PCT and have fully integrated IT communication with practices. It will be able to offer solutions to age-old problems. These solutions will include:

- advice for minor ailments to free up practice time

- integration of social services/primary care out-of-hours

- centralised booking for GP appointments

- 24-hour appointment cancellation service

- telephone translation service

- 'out-calling' to at-risk patients

NHS Direct will evolve to become part of primary care rather than a stand-alone service.

The walk-in centre will be an integral part of every primary care trust. It will need to be 'owned' by primary care. The walk-in centre will develop a multiplicity of roles. It will work as a safety net for the chaotic and underprivileged. It will operate as a 'health shop' for the locality. It will take redirected patients from A&E. It will be flexible enough to offer services according to the needs of the local population, such as tourists, the mobile mentally ill, commuters and those needing emergency contraception. The walk-in centre will be integrated into local primary care services. GP registration will be facilitated. Bilateral referral will take place. Access to primary care will be varied, flexible and integrated.

Structure

Primary care groups will evolve into primary care trusts. The list based practice will remain its foundation. Co-operation between practices will increase, with sharing of staff, equipment, and training. Practice based services will be extended. Enormous benefit will be gained by fully integrating, with health, key elements of social services, i.e. elderly, mental health, physical and learning disabilities.

The aims of *Saving Lives, Our Healthier Nation*[1] will only be achieved by better health education. Every practice will have its own linked/based health promotion worker. Education and information can be so much more effective if it is delivered 'from the community'.

The changes in the medical workforce will mean that fewer GPs opt for independent contractor status in singlehanded practices. This will be mirrored by a growth in salaried GPs, working in group practices. Each practice will have a separate contract held with the PCT. The role of the practice nurse will expand into disease monitoring, minor illness management, triage and sub-specialisation.

The expanding role of IT will extend our capacity. The NHS Net will allow access to clinical information held previously only in a medical library. **We will be able to book outpatients, operations and diagnostic tests from our practices. We may choose to consult either on e-mail or the Internet.**

The NHS will remain free at the point of health care delivery. We may have persuaded the electorate that an excellent health service is worth paying for and a hypothecated Health Tax may be in place.

We may need to form new partnerships to ensure effective delivery of health care. Many GPs have formed partnerships with private companies to deliver their out-of-hours service. This is a precedent that may develop further. PCTs may choose to form similar partnerships with the voluntary and private sectors to address fluctuations in hospital activity and short term increases in capability.

Conclusion

The changes I have outlined will create a new paradigm for services delivery. However, no one can predict the future and whatever system is in place, it must be prepared to change again.

A vision for the future is hidden within the mind of all practitioners in primary care. Once their visions are displayed, discussed and collated it will then feel much safer to grasp the opportunities that modernising primary care offers us.

References
1. Department of Health. *Saving Lives, Our Healthier Nation.* 1999.

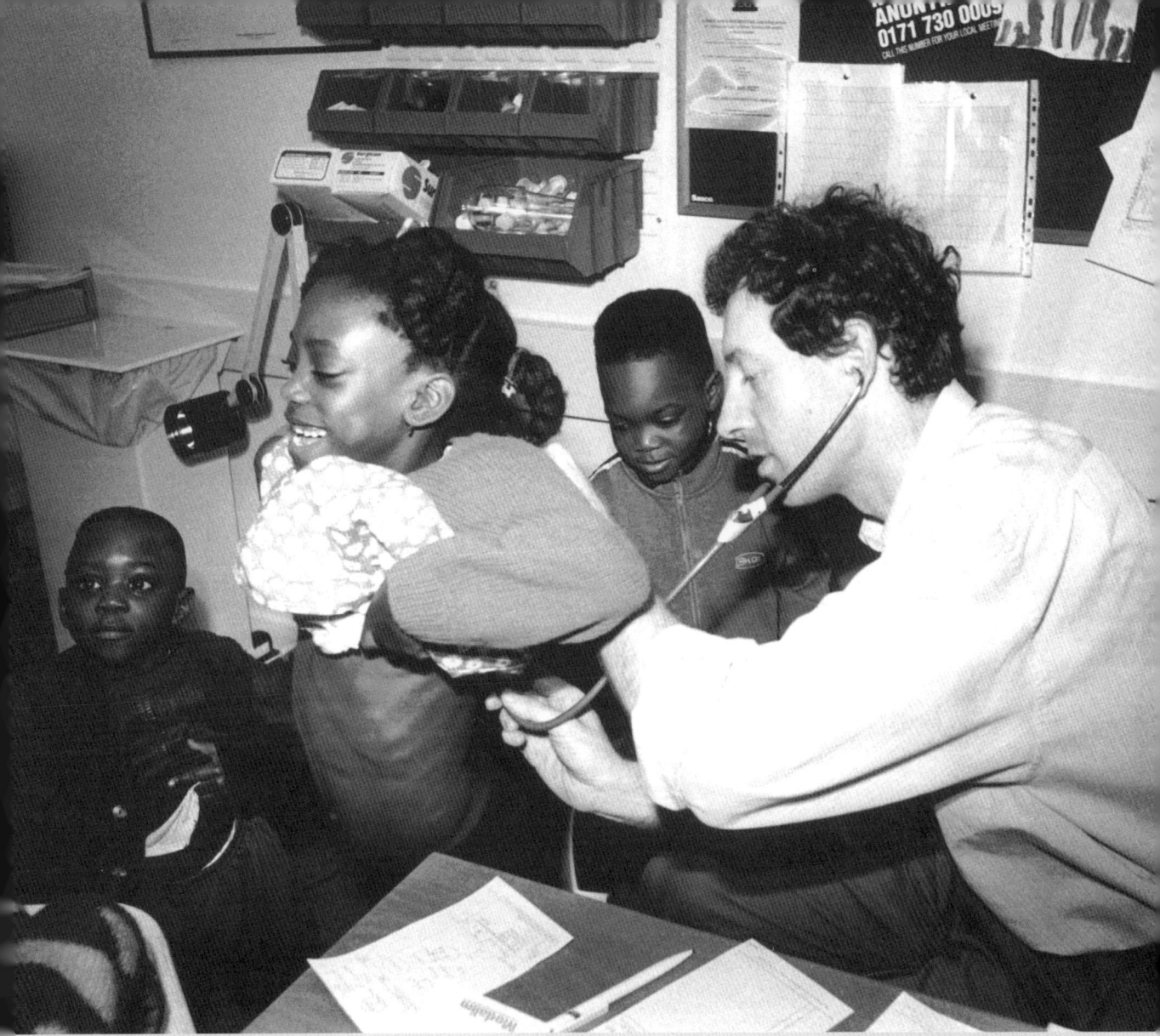

What will GPs be doing? Their role as generalists in terms of diagnosis will be increasingly in demand as secondary care specialisation continues unabated. Their potential as generalists will be helped by better and direct access to high technology investigations and greatly improved communication systems.

Vision 2

Co-operative working relationships

Michael Dixon
GP & Chair, NHS Alliance
Virtual PCG Board GP Member

THE WHITE PAPER *THE NEW NHS; MODERN, DEPENDABLE*[1] HAS SET THE SCENE FOR primary care over the next ten years. Any prediction of how things are likely to turn out will depend upon interpreting current Government thinking, observing how developments in primary care are presently working out and informed guess work.

One of the most positive aspects of primary care groups and trusts will be to bring GPs and other primary care professionals together in co-operative working relationships that never previously existed. The result will be better integrated primary care teams at the working face together with better division, integration and identification of responsibility between the different members of the primary care team such as GP, practice nurse, district nurse and health visitor.

Better co-operative working between GPs may lead to larger practices as they are more financially viable and easier to organise. Patients, however, prefer smaller practices, which will survive if they can form mutually supportive confederations that offer traditional patient care together with the advantages, in terms of services and division of responsibilities, of larger practices. Independent contractor and salaried status both offer advantages to professional, patient and the NHS, thus it is likely that the next ten years will see a 'mixed economy' of salaried and independent contractor GPs, both represented in each practice and possibly in a ratio of 50/50.

What will the GPs be doing? **Their role as generalists in terms of diagnosis will be increasingly in demand as secondary care specialisation continues unabated. Their potential as generalists will be helped by better and direct access to high technology investigations and greatly**

improved communication systems. Their role is likely to alter, however, in acute disease, where the nurse practitioner may become a valued asset providing easier access through triage and treatment of both minor acute illness and chronic conditions with clear protocols.

Within nursing itself, traditional barriers between district nurse, practice nurse, health visitor, school nurse and other branches are likely to fade as integrated nursing becomes the norm. Such changes will provide nurses with a prime position in localities, acting as key links for a number of patients and conditions. They will also have a major role in 'locality clinics' – such as musculoskeletal clinics or 'one-stop' headache clinics – which are likely to involve a primary care nurse and GP. Such 'integrated' services and clinics will ensure equity of access and resources in the locality and this form of locality-wide specialism is likely to prove more cost effective than super-specialism within each practice. In some areas, secondary care specialists and other professionals may devolve themselves from their bricks and mortar role and develop an increasingly primary care focus thus taking on a leading role in integrated care within the locality.

What about health? Primary care professionals will continue as holistic practitioners in their encounter with the individual patient but they will develop a new holistic role in looking after the health of the whole community. This role of primary care as an educator and leader within each community will require co-operation and integrated working with all health related agencies. As this happens, Health Improvement Programmes (HImPs) will cease to be the 'top down' creatures of the present and become amalgamated and edited versions ('himplets') derived through such co-operative working at grass roots level.

Demand management will become a major feature of primary care especially when this is seen as a means of ensuring equity and getting the best out of the pot rather than limited access because there is not enough money. Meanwhile corporate governance in primary care will create a new culture of change that will improve average standards and reduce lower standards of care. The determining factor will be the effectiveness of clinical leads in each practice and their ability to enthuse and inspire colleagues, who may feel threatened or even apathetic. They may also be the deciding factor in the success of the National Institute for Clinical Excellence and the National Service Frameworks.

This is how it will look, but how will it feel? Patients want good quality accessible care but the majority, especially over 65s, also want personal care. This is something well known to those who are ill and those who look after them. Patients will want care that is offered conveniently rather than 'convenience care'. Increasing 'patient power' within primary care groups/primary care trusts and cost effective evidence from HMOs will all counteract some of the current imperatives of evidence and cost effectiveness. A new balance will emerge between hard clinical evidence and holistic forces, cultural trends and traditions.

If patients and primary care professionals become alienated from each other then there will be a need for impersonal polyclinics and an NHS Direct-type service, which is divorced from traditional primary care. Where there are good relationships between primary care professionals and patients then both will develop local services to their mutual good without requiring further structural reorganisation. The 'responsible patient view' will increasingly dominate the pattern of services and patients will see themselves **less as individual consumers fighting for their rights and more as NHS citizens with a role in their own health and that of others,** as well as stakeholders in the shape of the future NHS.

The final factor will be the absolute level of resources. Primary care may find it more difficult than expected to stop the haemorrhage of resources into secondary care because of a number of factors including new technology and commitments made under the Private Finance Initiative. The ability of primary care to take over secondary care roles may prove limited, though integrated clinics will help. Primary care will need proper financing if it is to develop in its expanded role and if this happens then primary care professionals will be less inclined to want to retire early and patients will feel positively involved in the development of a better local health service. Indeed there is every reason to expect that primary care will become better, more accessible, more accountable and fairer as the new structures (primary care groups and primary care trusts) are both logical and robust. Nevertheless, you get what you pay for. Without proper financing, there is the danger that rhetoric and reality may never meet.

References
1. Department of Health. *The New NHS; Modern, Dependable.* 1997.

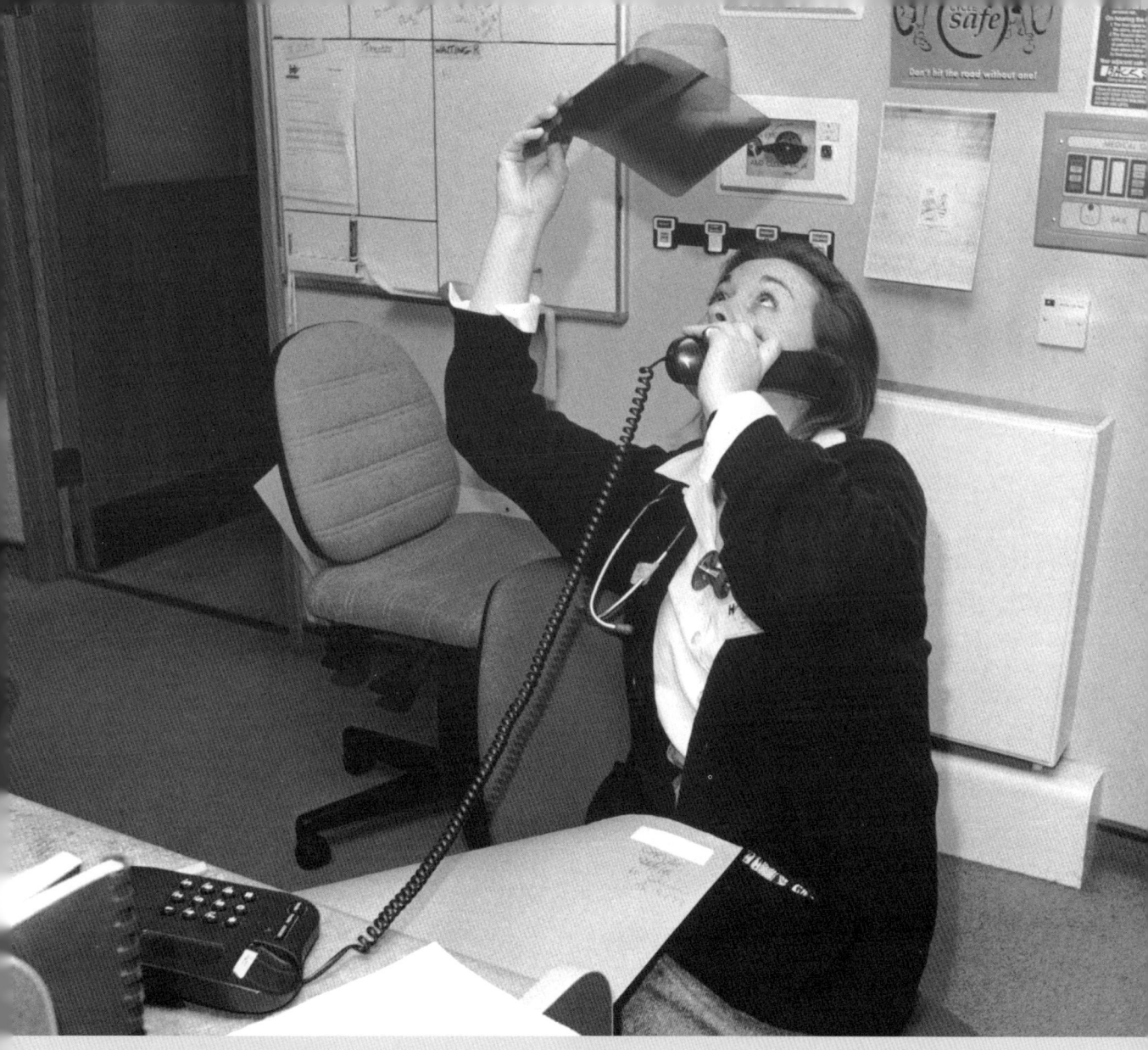

Medical professionals will work with the trust and other clinicians in the acute sector to devise innovative pathways of care.

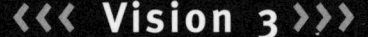

We need to guarantee uniform quality

Howard Freeman
GP & Co-chair, Nelson PCG
Virtual PCG Board GP Member

PREDICTING THE FUTURE FROM AFAR IS A BIT LIKE GENERAL PRACTICE; THERE IS A BASIS OF SCIENCE but it is overlaid with art. That art is a melange of many things, including personal perspective and current experience. **The future for primary care must be about delivering a service of uniform quality nationally but how that is achieved will depend very much on local circumstances.** My model is the one that will work for my population in suburban south west London. There will be others with similar models but there will also be near neighbours with very different approaches.

The underlying key theme for the NHS in 2004 will be providing the maximum amount of services possible of guaranteed uniform quality to local populations. The big parameters of what the NHS encompasses will be decided through a national debate, via a general election in which it is a major issue, and through the work of the National Institute for Clinical Excellence (NICE). Outliers will already have had their first visits from the Commission for Health Improvement, and clinical governance will encourage most health care professionals to deliver to an acceptable and uniform standard. Notwithstanding this approach there will be local variation as to exactly what the NHS Contract delivers, how it is delivered and what is excluded. The private sector will play a role, especially in continuing care and non-emergency work.

Locally all the primary care groups will evolve into primary care trusts (PCTs). For the first time all primary care professionals will be under the same management structure. Many GPs will go even further; through the mechanism of the Primary Care Act they will move from general medical services (GMS) to personal medical services (PMS) and their PCTs will hold their contract.

Some will decide that the financial elements of independent contractor status are no longer worth having. They will opt for an entire salaried service working alongside GPs who will be recruited and employed directly by the primary care trust to deliver service to well-defined patient groups. These will be groups who in the past have had problems engaging with traditional general practice, e.g. refugee populations.

Other doctors will begin to realise that their perspective in the past was from the wrong place and they too will leave acute trusts to join primary care trusts. The psychiatrists and the community mental health teams will lead this approach, followed rapidly by geriatricians and gynaecologists who will soon realise that their future lies in the community within reach and admission rights to local acute trusts. Many of the medical professionals will be quick to join the new multidisciplinary partnerships with GPs. Together they will negotiate their contracts with the trusts and **they will be able to work with the trust and other clinicians in the acute sector to devise innovative pathways of care.** The primary care doctors will often hold the budgets for these pathways as they will be better at being the gatekeepers to services than their hospital colleagues.

Similarly, in the nursing field, practice nurses will be quick to realise that they need to leave the employment of GPs and move directly to the employment of the primary care trust to ensure they have appropriate professional support, education, and training, and to take advantage of nurse clinical governance.

Clinical governance will be the key vehicle used to improve the quality of poorly performing professionals in the community and to ensure consistency of standards. It will move rapidly from looking at financial outliers to using more sophisticated performance indicators as IT develops. Increasingly the professionals within the trusts will respond to clinical governance. There will be the downside that improving quality will have significant cost implications for the trust. These will not just be direct costs but will include indirect costs such as the increasing need for professionals to have protected time for continuing professional development and retraining. In the light of continuing shortages of primary care professionals, increasingly tasks will be devolved to non-professionals who will be trained to deliver one specific task.

Following the evaluation of practice based services, decisions will be made about which services it is appropriate to deliver at practice level and which services need to be delivered to the wider population of the primary care trust. Decisions will be made as to which sets of premises need further development and how the finance will be raised via private public–partnership to achieve this. Some tough decisions will also be made about which premises are no longer needed for the delivery of primary care within the trust's patch. Negotiations will result in the purchase of these premises and the relocation of the professionals who work in them. The trust hospital site will be the setting for many of these additional services as well as for a whole range of other primary care professionals who have admitting rights to all the local acute trusts. As part of the redevelopment of the site a full range of diagnostic facilities will be built in and where it is not practical for these to be on site there will be telemedicine links to other local sites.

While the hospital site will have no beds of its own, a nursing home will be built on the site, working closely with the day hospital facility. The nursing home will specialise not only in the elderly infirm but also in the elderly mentally ill, and it will offer step down and rehabilitation facilities for acutely ill young people discharged from acute units. This process will be facilitated by the merger of the trust with the local authority social services department. For the first time, the trust will be able to take an overview not only of health services but also of personal social services. Integrating the service delivery teams on the ground – especially the generalist district nursing service with the home care services – and making these teams self-managing, will allow the new unified health and social services budgets to be operationally maximised.

The trust board will guide the development of the trust from its early days. Until its abolition it will relate to its local health authority but will then relate to both its local borough council, who will be responsible for the local delivery of health care policy, and to the Greater London Authority who will hold the responsibility for the strategic direction of health policy in London. The board will actively discuss merger proposals between itself and two of its adjacent PCT neighbours. It will also become one of the leading players in the discussions between the two remaining local acute trusts about their merger and the relocation of many of the acute trust services out into the primary care trusts and the community. In its annual report the board will be delighted to announce that using its consumer focus groups the level of satisfaction with the trust's services has reached an all time high of over 95 per cent. Complaints to the trust about service delivery and the health care professionals who delivered the service will drop to an all time low.

From the perspective of 2004 it will be a somewhat daunting experience to look down the mountain that has been climbed by primary care in the preceding decade. In 1994 the first steps along the road through GP fundholding had only just begun. Few people would have expected it to lead to this point within a decade. Even more challenging will be looking up the mountain at the climb for the next decade.

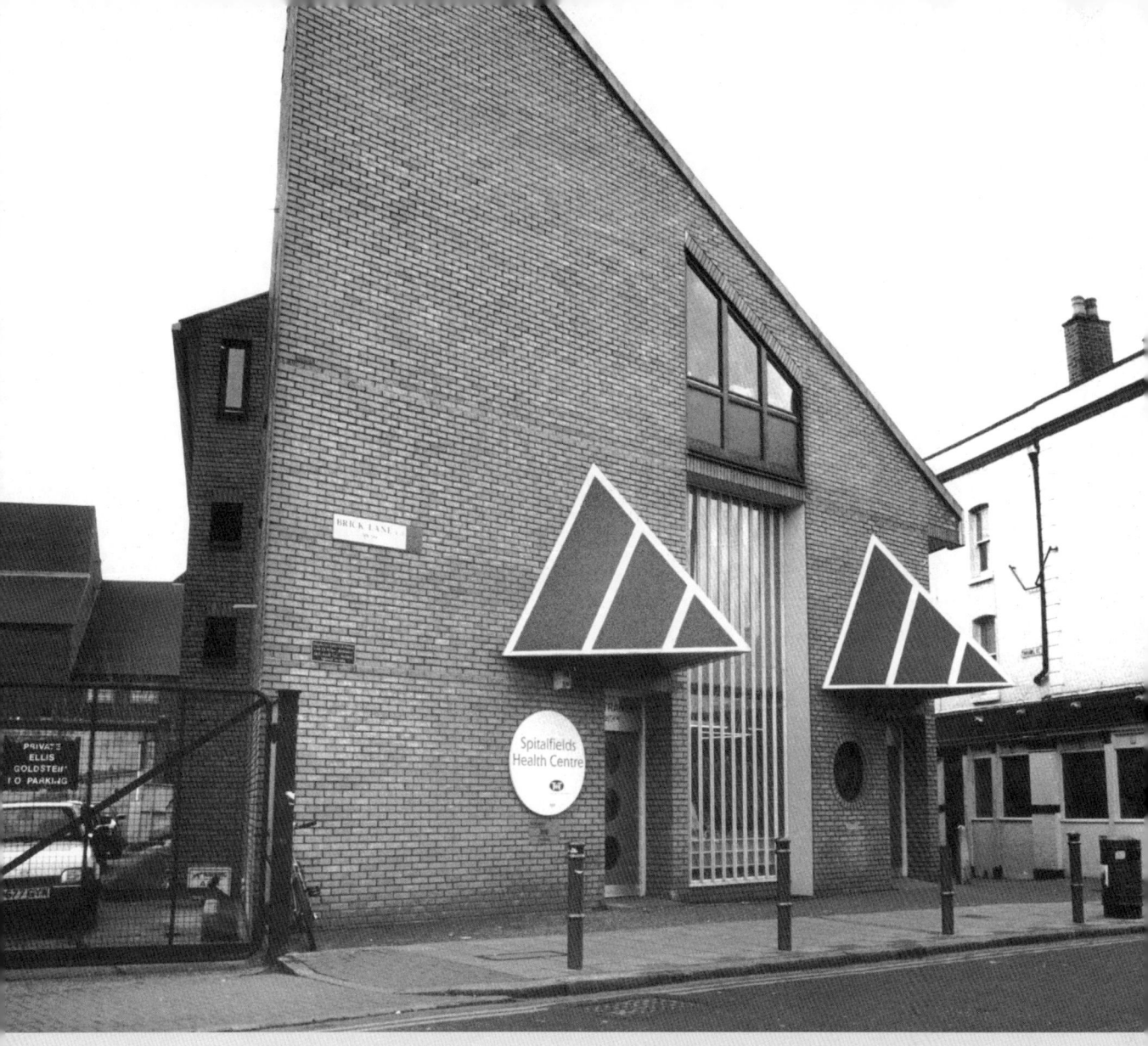

Decisions will be made as to which sets of premises need further development and how the finance will be raised via public–private partnership to achieve this. Some tough decisions will also be made about which premises are no longer needed for the delivery of primary care within the trust's area.

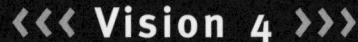

The impact of information technology on health care

Paul Cundy
GP & Chair, IM&T subcommittee of BMA's General Practioners Committee
Virtual PCG Board GP Member

PRIMARY CARE GROUPS EVOLVED VIA PRIMARY CARE TRUSTS INTO PRIMARY CARE ORGANISATIONS (PCOs). This was largely completed by 2005. The further development of NHS Direct, walk-in centres, NICE, online services and the increasing use of Internet technologies blew apart the traditional linkage between a patient and their registered GP. Now, in 2009, patients are registered with a PCO not a GP and consult a variety of health care professionals (HCPs). HCPs are a generic grouping of what we used to call GPs – in all their forms, full-time, part-time, partners, assistants, salaried partners and plain employees – but also nurses, health visitors, mental and social health workers and all the other professions allied to medicine (PAMs).

This change was enabled and accelerated by the use of information technology and the refinement of information management skills. The realisation that an electronic patient record can be operated as a distributed record between a variety of different sites and providers has reflected **the increasing tendency for patients to determine where, when and from whom they seek their health care.** Distributing a patient's lifelong electronic health care record over the Internet only became possible with increasing data transmission speeds and the provision of effectively free fixed connections. A distributed electronic health care record consists of a string of linked web pages or sites, each containing components of the patient's health records. When the patient consults an HCP they browse the relevant parts of the patient's history. The record of that consultation can then be appended to the previous records via complex and automatic links not dreamed of in 1999.

Each HCP has local possession and ownership of 'their' contribution to that patient's record, but at the same time all the records from all HCPs are available for present and future consultations.

In 2009, HCPs are not the only significant contributors to a patient's health record. The proliferation of near patient devices means that every household will have a vast array of telemetric equipment. The development of universal use connection (UUC) has enabled any electronic device to communicate with any other and with no physical links. A palm-sized optical biochemistry device makes a link, does the analysis, and downloads the results automatically and in seconds from the patient's bedroom.

Real time predictive interchange between your own personally tailored monitoring software and these new devices means that your health is continually monitored. **Regular checks and tests are planned and adapted in the same way that cars inform their drivers when they need servicing.** HCPs are automatically alerted if you default or if any reading varies from your personal norm. If you normally go to the toilet at 8 a.m. and have fallen on the way to the bathroom, real time predictive interchange will be warning that something may be wrong. The sophistication of electrodigital diagnostics (EDD) means that nearly every test once available only in hospital is now available in the home. Non-invasive imaging has been developed to reflect physical, physiological and metabolic activity.

Virtual sensing technologies enable emergency care to be delivered by devices that can crawl into nooks and crannies where a human would not fit.

Clinical decision support systems such as those first brought to the UK by NHS Direct and the co-operative movement in the late 1990s soon found general acceptance among professionals and within a few years they were extended beyond diagnostic advice to treatment management.

It was soon realised that triage nurses were merely expensive typists. **The development of direct interfaces where callers complete voice-driven online questionnaires linked to their electronic health records means that for certain conditions patients will be able to generate their own prescriptions for a range of agreed drugs.** This process is the so-called SOC (self online consultation).

Developing the distributed database electronic record will free up the clinicians' dependence on technology. There is no longer any need for a clinician to have anything other than a hand-held browsing device (HHBD) operating without wires through the UUC.

Of course all these developments only became acceptable with increased sophistication of security arrangements backed up by appropriate legislation. Dual key encryption gave way to biometric patient identifier keys. These were generated by the patient and HCP's combined fingerprints, but these were found to be forgeable.

The development of real time pupillary reaction measurement (PRM) provided us with a patient identifier that is almost impossible to falsify. It only needs revision in certain infrequent circumstances. When the patient consults the physician, a quick squint at the pupil scanner is all that is required to unlock their record for the duration of the consultation. Proxies operate for those unable to consent by virtue of age or other disability and of course every patient has an area of their record accessible to any verified member of the emergency services for basic data.

In all it is a very different world apart from one thing – acronyms abound!

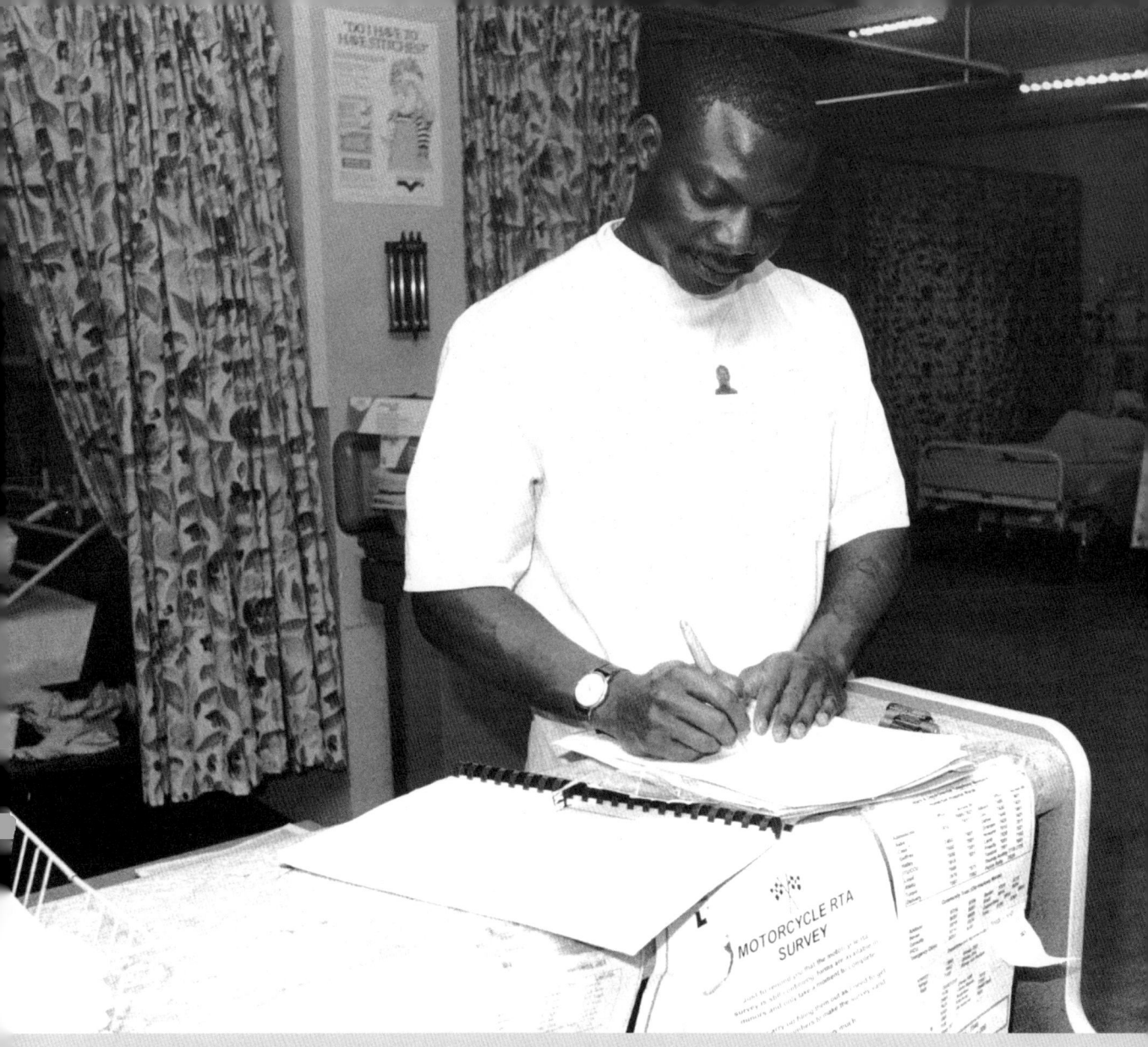

Intermediate care will be seen not to be intermediate but rather an integral part of primary care, funded and managed by the primary care trust (even if the service is not staffed exclusively by primary care professionals). The challenge to, and the re-design of, secondary care will gather pace both in resource utilisation and clinical appropriateness.

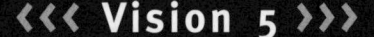

New models of primary care

David Colin-Thomé
GP & Director of Primary Care, NHS Executive London
Virtual PCG Board GP Member

IN AN ORGANISATION AS CONSERVATIVE AND COLLECTIVIST AS THE NATIONAL HEALTH SERVICE, IT MAY be too much to expect that by 2009, even with the added catalyst of the Millennium, significant *behavioural* change will occur (although there may be significant *structural* change). Nonetheless there remains a continuing hope that the NHS may be about to witness completely different patterns of service delivery. The magnitude of change that will have taken place by 2009 is therefore doubly difficult to predict. My vision for primary care in 2009 assumes that its existing strengths and the wider demographic and cultural drivers acting on it will, together, provide the catalyst for change.

Traditional general practice has delivered care that is personal, co-ordinated and continuous as well as providing a 'gatekeeper function' for entry to other types of care. There are well documented variations in general practice performance but the general practice system, together with the cheapness of the National Health Service continue, when viewed from abroad, to be the most envied parts of our National Health Service. These are a consequence both of the gatekeeper role and the registered general practice population and should, other things being equal, continue to make general practice attractive to successive governments. Accordingly, such a health system, ensuring as it does a cheap yet comprehensive and personalised care service would, at first glance, seem to need little change. And yet, despite the popularity of general practice with the vast majority of patients, this envied system may be difficult to sustain, as the utility that patients place on such a personalised service decreases. Empirical trend evidence, confirmed by the NHS User Survey, is that **patients increasingly place greater value on easy access to care above a long term relationship with their 'personal' doctor,** and such doctors are in any case increasingly difficult to recruit at a time when patient demand has increased.

New models of primary care

Responding to such pressures, new models of primary care are beginning to emerge:

GP hospitals: these will be *'purpose-built or housed in existing buildings with no overnight beds, housing 50–80 better remunerated doctors who provide, in addition to family medicine, specialist outpatient clinics, day surgery and comprehensive diagnostic tests. These GPs will work closely with hospital consultants with a much enlarged multidisciplinary team and a 24-hour emergency service. No longer will individual practice premises be dotted around the town ... rather there will be an emergence of a much more dispersed and accessible Primary Care service with "health shops" in places like schools, malls, hotels and work places'*.[1]

Practice based contract systems: the move to practice based contract systems, as manifested at the present time in the personal medical services pilots that have already taken 6 per cent of general practices outside of the traditional personal remuneration system.

Law firm type models: with both partners and salaried professionals who are not all doctors.

Private models of care: where GPs either charge patients or have hybrid systems of private and state care (although this last model may not be culturally acceptable in the United Kingdom).

My vision of primary care

It is often said that to predict the future one needs to look to current best practice and, on that basis, my view is that while the practice with its registered population will remain the bedrock of primary health care, it will only do so if primary health care workers are prepared to play a more responsive, wider and proactive role as a *resource* to their communities.

Continuity of personal care and small rather than large practices remain important to the NHS's end user, as demonstrated by the 80 per cent satisfaction rate for general practice in the recent NHS User Survey. In my vision, such care attributes need to be retained, while recognising that achieving personal care and increased accessibility may mean that continuity of care rather than continuity of carer[2] may become the predominant model. Linked information systems will ensure continuity through comprehensive information bases. Already, advice and first contact care for patients do not necessarily come from general practice, demonstrating the continuity of care rather than carer model. Indeed, the pharmacist could already be described as a model of a walk-in centre, a model acceptable to general practice although, sadly, information is not often interchanged. The future would see collaboration between daytime and out-of-hours general practice services, minor injury units, walk-in centres, pharmacists and NHS Direct to make a coherent responsive whole. Such collaboration could be facilitated and overseen by primary care trusts.

The practice's role would be as a first contact point for patients who choose that option, the point of continuity of care for episodic illnesses, as well as ensuring continuity and co-ordination of care through care management for chronic disease sufferers. **The first contact clinician in the practice is as likely to be a nurse as a doctor but will still need to be perceived as a personal carer for the patient.**

The practice may also adopt a public health population perspective along with its important personal care function. Such public health initiatives could be led by health visitors and school nurses forming alliances with environmental health officers, and include health needs assessment, anticipatory care in all its different modes, interagency working, community development as well as clinical governance. Professor Jenny Popey at Salford University is currently exploring such an approach.

In my vision, by 2009 primary care trusts will develop to be the integrators and re-designers of clinical care, certainly to the level of secondary care provision. Intermediate care will be seen not to be intermediate but rather an integral part of primary care, funded and managed by the trust (even if the service is not staffed exclusively by primary care professionals). The challenge to, and the re-design of, secondary care will gather pace both in resource utilisation and clinical appropriateness. Many consultant colleagues, in particular geriatricians, psychiatrists and paediatricians together with their teams could well, in real or virtual form, become part of the primary care trust, using the hospital as a facility together with their GP and nursing colleagues. A similar integrated approach will have been developed with social services.

A new primary care beckons, encompassing the attributes of traditional general practice, varied but information-linked (joined up in the current parlance) first contact points for patients, radically re-designed hospital care funded by primary care trusts and a public health focus that links health care to the wider health agenda to address the social determinants of health. Primary care trusts will be the commissioners of such primary care. Such a vision of primary care will in itself require vision, strong leadership and a new, more facilitative management style if it is to flourish. Delivering this agenda will need a significant mind set change, not least the acceptance of an overt accountability of primary care to the public in general and patients in particular – a significant challenge, but not an impossible one!

References
1. L McMahon, *Personal Communication*, 1999.
2. L Haggard, *Personal Communication*, 1999.

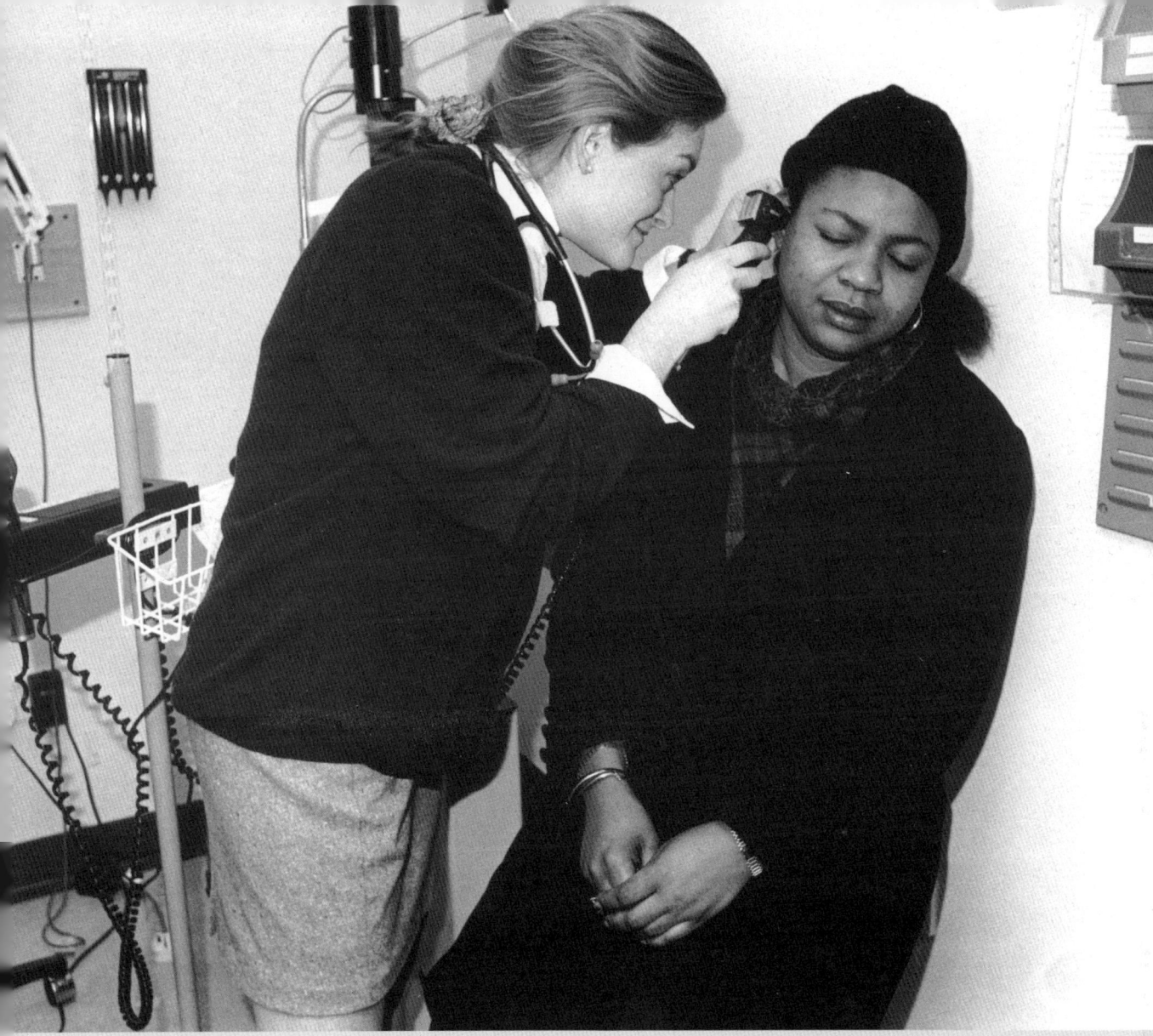

Patients increasingly place greater value on easy access to care above a long term relationship with their 'personal' doctor.

Shifting professional roles in the primary health care team

Toby Lipman
GP & Research Training Fellow, NHS Executive Northern & Yorkshire
Virtual PCG Board GP Member

AT THE FOUNDATION OF THE NHS, MOST GPS WORKED IN SMALL PRACTICES, OFTEN SINGLEHANDED with perhaps a receptionist and the GP's spouse as the only staff. They had few clinical resources by today's standards and were expected to refer 'serious' illness to hospital specialists (although they were involved in the delivery of babies). They thus acted primarily as gatekeepers to secondary care. Their present role and training have evolved from an ideal, defined in the late 1960s, in which: '...[the GP] accepts the responsibility for making an initial decision on every problem his patient may present to him, consulting with specialists when he thinks it appropriate to do so'.[1]

Since the 1960s group practices have become the norm and have increased in size. The primary health care team, consisting of practice nurses, community nurses, midwives, health visitors, receptionists, secretaries, practice managers, counsellors, physiotherapists and others has expanded around GPs. Despite this, GPs have experienced an increase in workload and stress in recent years, and, after a brief burst of enthusiasm in the late 1970s and early 1980s, general practice has become less popular as a specialty.

The reasons for this include increased demand and expectation, and the growing fear of complaints and litigation. **Doctors are no longer assumed to 'know best' and patients are less willing to accept what they say without question.** There is increased suspicion of orthodox medicine and many patients are choosing alternative therapies. Paradoxically, the last decade has seen a revolution in medical science, and has increased opportunities to treat serious illness in primary care – illness that once was either untreatable, or needed specialist care in hospital. GPs can now have open access to almost all diagnostic tests (in the 1950s patients often had to be referred for some blood tests, never mind X-rays) and can prescribe effective medication for conditions such as heart failure, duodenal ulcer, enlarged prostate and many other formerly 'hospital' diseases.

However, most patients going to see their GPs do not have serious illnesses. One of the most common of GPs' complaints is that seeing patients with 'trivial' conditions prevents them from being able to tackle the minority of 'serious' health problems. GPs often talk about 'educating' patients not to bother them with coughs and colds and the like, and the establishment of telephone triage and NHS Direct are responses to this perceived problem. But the problem is structural, and lies in GPs' historical role as the centre of the primary health care team, and their implied obligation to respond to any and all of their patients' needs. This obligation is now impossible to fulfil, and perhaps counter-productive.

Access to the NHS, except in some emergency situations, is normally through the GP (the 'gatekeeper' function). The GP traditionally either treats the patient's condition, delegates treatment to another member of the team, or refers the patient to hospital. Often he or she acts as a conduit to other professionals or services rather than as an active clinician. In other cases, particularly where patients present with emotional or social problems, medical interventions are not beneficial and the GP must function as a combination of counsellor, social worker, psychologist and priest. When minor illnesses are also taken into account, much, perhaps the major part, of GPs' workload requires them either not to intervene medically (such as in self-limiting minor illness), or to advise about non-medical health related problems.

Illich pointed out the dangers of 'social iatrogenesis' or the 'medicalisation of life'.[2] By this, he meant that people were losing control over basic aspects of life and health, from birth to death, which were being expropriated by the medical establishment. The paradox of general practice is that it was the first medical specialty to take these criticisms seriously and advocate a Patient-centred approach to health care. **By placing GPs at the centre of primary care it encourages a medical response to non-medical (even if health-related) problems such as unhappiness, social deprivation, unfitness, and everyday minor ailments (with the hurtful implication that if the problem is not 'medical' it is not important).** At the same time, modern developments in medicine make the effective management of serious disease in primary care an attainable goal.

The time has come for a shifting of roles in primary care, and the removal of GPs from their central position. The development of nurse practitioners, telephone triage and health care web sites brings an opportunity to provide patients with a service more appropriate to their everyday needs, which will rarely encompass serious disease. Primary care groups (and later trusts) will employ a range of health professionals such as physiotherapists, osteopaths, counsellors and therapists, and must develop means of identifying who can most benefit each patient. Health care web sites and telephone advice will help patients to choose whom they need to see, and access them directly. For example, if you have back pain it is much more sensible to make an appointment with a physiotherapist in the first instance than with a GP. The GP's pastoral role will be shared (as it already is in practice) with other members of the team.

GPs will see a smaller proportion of patients registered with their team compared with today, but most of these will have significant medical diagnostic or therapeutic problems. Consultations will be longer, and informed by the practice of evidence-based medicine, *'...a process of life-long, self-directed learning in which caring for our own patients creates the need for clinically important information about diagnosis, prognosis, therapy and other clinical and health care issues.'*[3] They will routinely search electronic databases for evidence to inform their management, critically appraise it and use it to determine the most up to date and effective choices of clinical interventions. They will play a leading part in running educational activities within the primary health care team, in clinical audit and other quality assurance activities. The organisation of the team will emphasise holistic health care, while ensuring that patients with medical conditions receive optimal assessment, advice and treatment.

References

1. Royal College of General Practitioners. *The future general practitioner: learning and teaching.* London: BMJ, 1972.
2. Illich I. *Limits to medicine. Medical nemesis: the expropriation of health.* London: Penguin, 1976.
3. Sackett DL, Richardson WS, Rosenberg W, Haynes RB. *Evidence-based medicine. How to Practise and Teach EBM.* London: Churchill Livingstone, 1997.

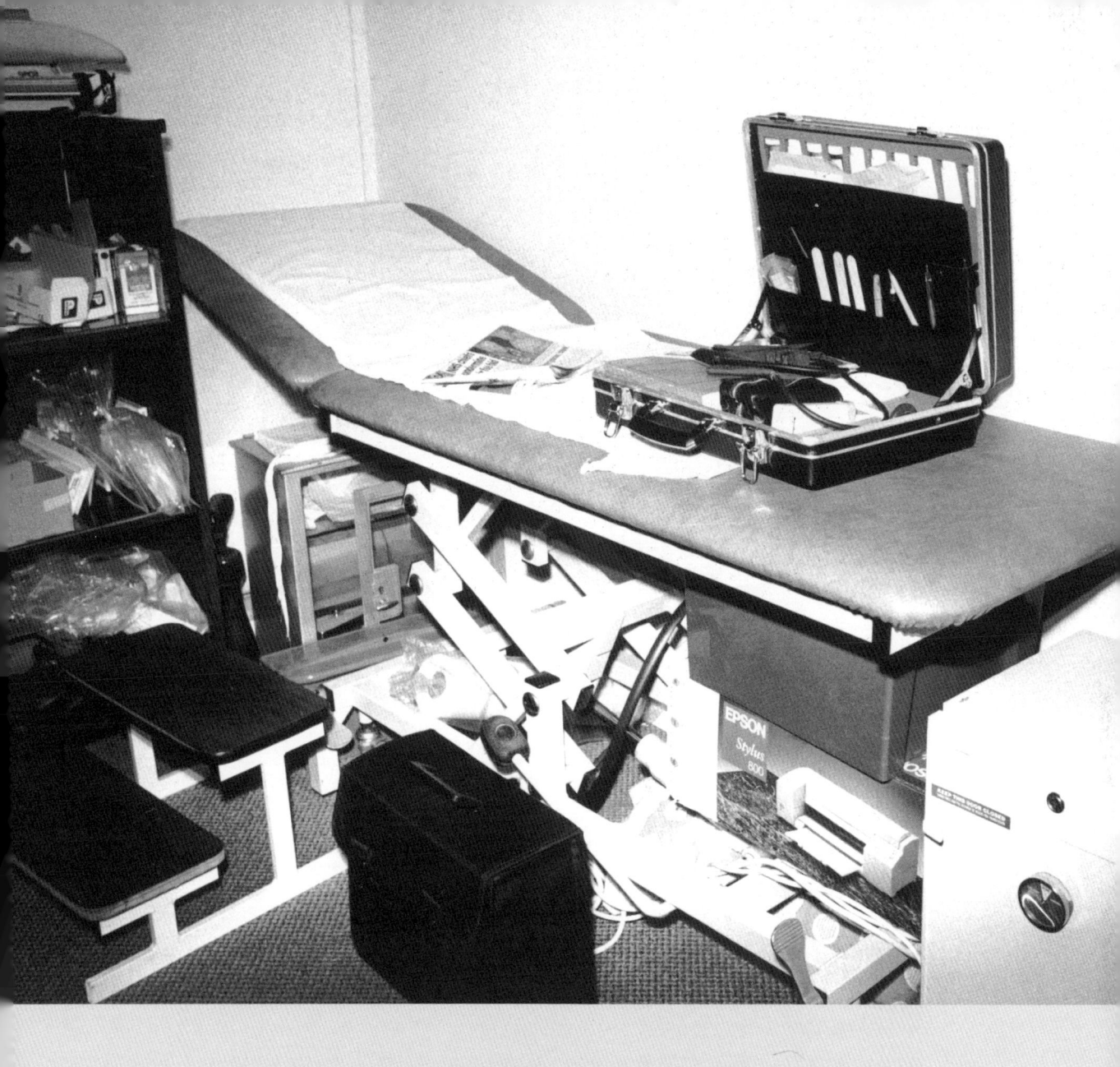

By placing GPs at the centre of primary care it encourages a medical response to non-medical (even if health-related) problems such as unhappiness, social deprivation, unfitness, and everyday minor ailments (with the hurtful implication that if the problem is not 'medical' it is not important).

Vision 7

The best care within finite resources

Gill Fraser
GP & Medical Director, Northumbria Healthcare NHS Trust
Virtual PCG Board GP Member

Primary care is well liked by patients and plays a vital role in the NHS. It is admired all over the world and provides continuity of care for individuals and their families. However, it is in danger of losing its way. On the one hand it is seen as increasingly inflexible in a world of customer-friendly round-the-clock services and on the other it is used inappropriately by people as the answer to all their problems. How can we preserve the best that primary care has to offer while managing ever-increasing demand?

Patient access to primary care will have to be managed. Many people consult inappropriately for minor or acute illness better dealt with elsewhere. Firstly this is due to lack of clarity for people as to how best to enter the health system. Primary care has been regarded as the 'gatekeeper' for the NHS, protecting secondary services from unnecessary contacts. This is entirely valid for hospital care but the primary health care team has become the screen for all access into the system. People are simply not clear as to how to seek help and are all too often advised to 'see your GP'. Secondly it has been important to raise awareness of the potential for minor symptoms to herald serious illness. People have a much lower threshold for seeking health advice than they did a generation ago, and we must accept the increase in demand to enable us to intervene early when it is important to do so.

Triage processes like NHS Direct will be the key to directing patients to the right person, in the right place at the right time. Safe, well-tried algorithms consistent across the country and in front of all 'urgent' access to primary care (both in and out-of-hours) will ensure an appropriate outcome tailored to each individual. Most contacts with primary care will be by telephone and at the end of the conversation the patient will have an arranged plan – be it the imminent arrival of an ambulance or an appointment next Tuesday at 6.30 p.m. with a physiotherapist. Outcomes will involve all disciplines and agencies, so a social services visit, a dental appointment, a discussion with a community pharmacist or a consultation with an occupational psychologist will all be equally available. The implications for joint thinking across agencies and professional groups are major, as are those for the linking of information technology.

The other access point for patients to the NHS is through A&E departments and this is an increasing problem where primary care is failing to meet demand. The same arguments apply but people are usually already in the department rather than at the end of the telephone. Using the same principle of triage, but this time face-to-face, consistent outcomes can be arranged for patients. In time people will use the telephone first before committing themselves to a journey that may be to the wrong place.

It may be that patients with an acute problem will choose to be seen by the nearest available primary care provider, for example the most convenient appointment at any surgery across a PCG or a primary care team based at the A&E department. This is already the accepted norm for out-of-hours care.

Introduction of clinically validated triage delivered in a Patient-centred way will free primary health care teams to do the job at which they excel – the continuing care of patients with complex needs, chronic disease management in its widest sense.

For primary care to achieve this extended role, staff of all professions will work across traditional practice boundaries to provide high quality evidence-based care. 'Hospital' consultants of all disciplines will indeed consult – providing clinical leadership, education, introducing new developments and individual advice to primary care staff. **Outpatient clinics will cease to exist. Patients will access hospital investigation or treatment direct. Hospital stays will be short with care being delivered in local community hospitals or at home. Regular telephone contact with patients to help them to manage their illness and to spot warning signs will become accepted.** Skill mix will determine the best person for the job, with changing roles envisaged for all health professionals.

Standards will be set, monitored and enforced by evidence-based contracts between PCGs/PCTs, hospital providers and health authorities. Patients need to be reassured that they will receive the same high standard of care wherever they live.

Traditional primary and secondary care boundaries will disappear. Already GPs contribute to the clinical strategy of our trust and work with clinical directors and trust managers on joint development. Common information is standard and a GP in each PCG shares responsibility for the community budget and the management of the community hospital. Likewise, hospital staff are increasingly involved in primary care activities. Pathways of care determine best treatment. Clinical excellence to foster evidence-based practice, quality audit and active research and development is a shared agenda.

Joint training and rotation of posts through primary, community and secondary care will be necessary to develop common understanding and maintain standards. This should include all disciplines, and shared modules for undergraduate training between nurses, professions allied to medicine (PAMs), medical students, social workers and health care managers should be available.

There are many areas of the NHS where shared information is vital. Apart from the obvious benefits to patient care a common approach to clinical governance, health and safety, risk management, human resource strategy, workforce planning and occupational health will provide a safe and flexible environment for staff.

Health promotion will play an increasing role in primary care. Multidisciplinary links with schools, colleges and universities, training centres and the workplace will develop. Joint work with other agencies, including the voluntary sector, to encourage healthier lifestyles for all will become more important. Support for a growing elderly population will become a major issue.

Primary care will also need to consider how to consult with the public and to involve their patients in decision-making. Resources are finite and how we choose to allocate them is of concern to us all. At present people believe in the future of primary care – it is up to us to maintain that belief and to deliver a service that our patients trust and value.

Brian Fisher
GP & Vice Chair, South Lewisham PCG
Virtual PCG Board GP Member

PUBLIC INVOLVEMENT AND PATIENT-CENTRED CARE ARE CENTRAL TO THE NEW NHS, BUT IT REMAINS singularly vague on these topics. This may be because of the complexity of issues and techniques involved. They will result in a shift of power away from the professions, for which we are unprepared.

Accountability, sharing decision-making and planning result in professionals relinquishing control in favour of lay people. This will require a shift not only in structures and organisation, but also in the mind-set of all of us in the NHS.

This paper sketches a Patient-centred primary care. It is critically dependent on PCGs creating the culture and pushing forward a programme of change – they contain the necessary elements, they can make it happen.

The one to one consultation

Patients want their bodies and minds treated with respect. They and their families want information about their condition and its management given in ways appropriate to their language and educational level. They want enough time to ask questions and have them answered. They want their condition taken seriously. A minority want to take decisions about their medical care.

A number of approaches might support these needs. Patients may have automatic access to their records, computerised or paper – browsing through them in the waiting room, correcting inaccuracies and asking questions. They will have access, from the GP, to their hospital electronic records. They can use terminals in waiting and consulting rooms to gain personalised information about their condition, with printable data about management options including complementary and drug therapies. This data will be evidence-based, include patient defined outcomes and explain where knowledge is inadequate. It will be routine to return to the professional, doctor or nurse to discuss issues after this data has been absorbed.

The professionals in the consultation will see themselves as facilitating the patient or parent in coming to conclusions that suit them. Young people will be spoken to directly where possible, and will be able to access primary care on their own.

In addition, as a result of community activity linked with the practice, there will be a range of support groups available locally. Social issues that impact on individuals will be seen as a prime responsibility of the practice. There will be excellent links with housing, trades unions and the local trades council.

The Patient-centred practice – what it might look like

Patients in urgent need will be able to see a professional, often a nurse, within half a day. It will be possible to book appointments of variable lengths, and communicate with the practice by e-mail and fax. It will be clear what tests are being taken, and there will be procedures for receiving results and explanations about their meaning. Patients will carry their own health data on card or disc, readable anywhere in the world.

There will be free exchange between local groups, people and practices through an independent community development organisation. This will have three tasks – to develop low-tech services defined and designed by local people, to engage local users in needs assessments and recommendations for improvements, and to work with the primary care trust (PCT), neighbourhoods and local authorities in implementing such changes.

Practice GPs will be mainly salaried and, although incentives for innovation and development will remain, the organisation will see itself as accountable to the local community through a locality council consisting of local authority, lay people elected through the community development organisation, CHC, industry and PCG/PCT reps. Users' recommendations will be debated at council meetings. Interviewing panels will include lay people.

This will require a significant change in approach and culture supported by the PCT with incentives and education, including a 'Patients as Teachers' programme in which users, in a two-stage process, define good practice from their points of view and then train professionals, in facilitated meetings.

Primary care, the community and the primary care trust

An increase in social investment will lead to substantial health benefit across disease groups. A supportive environment is a public health issue.

The PCT will see one of its main roles as supporting local people in creating a better health service, viewing health in a broad context.

For instance, working with housing, employment, community development, public health and mental health services, the PCT might offer a comprehensive efficient service that will allow medical and social responses to mental illness. Elderly services commissioned jointly with social services will ensure a single point of contact for each elderly housebound person, with efficient services doing what they promise with flexibility and care. In response to young peoples' wishes, PCTs will employ youth health advisors to develop outreach services to encourage young people to use primary care appropriately. They will liaise with schools, developing an educational programme defined by the young people themselves and encouraging local practices to develop youth centred approaches.

The PCT will use community development as its link with the complex world of community groups and voluntary organisations. Allowing rapid responses to PCTs' needs for community views and using eclectic methods to garner ideas from local people, it will have a place on the board but remain independent from it. In this way, a notion of accountability will be created.

Education and clinical governance

Seeing patients, particularly those with chronic disease, as experts on aspects of their condition will allow a more holistic educational approach. Patients will prove themselves to be effective in changing clinical practice.

For each Health Improvement Programme (HImP) topic, user defined outcomes will set part of the agenda against which practices will be monitored, sometimes by users themselves, perhaps as 'mystery shoppers'. For instance, a high priority for patients is that side-effects of medication be explained. This could be monitored by users of medication, perhaps with the help of the local medical audit and research group.

Localities will be taught research techniques for involving users at different levels and linking with existing groups. Each practice will be encouraged to work with a different key patient group each year, for instance patients with heart disease, or those with diabetes.

Conclusion

PCG/PCTs can deliver on this kind of agenda, despite the obvious organisational and emotional changes required. The examples used here are neither speculative nor expensive. Most of the initiatives described are based on examples under development or in place somewhere in the UK or elsewhere. User involvement offers a significant step forward in both the form and content of health care.

‹‹‹ Vision 9 ›››

NICE's role in unlocking potential

Andrew Dillon
Chief Executive, National Institute for Clinical Excellence (NICE)
Virtual PCG Board Chief Executive

IF THERE IS A SENSE, IN 1999, OF UNREALISED POTENTIAL IN PRIMARY CARE, HOW MIGHT THIS change by 2009? And in what way might the National Institute for Clinical Excellence (NICE), launched with so much prospect itself at the beginning of that period, contribute to unlocking that potential?

A range of forces for change will influence the development of primary care. The aspirations and abilities of clinicians themselves, the enthusiasm of patients for conveniently located services in comfortably scaled settings and the ability of technology to bring diagnosis and decisions about treatment – into the surgery or the home – are some of the key drivers.

Comparing primary care now with its future will see much gained, but some familiar things lost too. Access to first line advice will be much quicker – immediate for those with the confidence and ability to use web-based and telephone advice systems which will be heavily promoted by Our Health – the new state–citizen partnership that will evolve from the old NHS. **Initial diagnosis will be fast and accurate, driven by guidelines and decisions trees developed by NICE, but it will be less personal.** The telephone advice system operators will be confident, concerned and friendly, with many, by then, trained specifically to operate diagnosis software, backed up by clinical professionals. But they will be different every time, without the ability to develop a relationship with those who need to access the service regularly. The system will have the ability to monitor critical indicators – over the phone directly or through the web. Our Health will give patients the opportunity to take more responsibility for the management of their care by offering informed choices – and there will be a gentle pressure for patients to consider and exercise these choices. **The new partnership will bring with it an expectation of active patient interest and involvement,** where there is a reasonable possibility of this happening.

Practitioners

The practitioners will be both familiar and different. They will be familiar from their basic training and labels, as physiotherapists or nurses or doctors. They will be different in what they do and the extent to which they take responsibility, with patients, for the management of care. **The dominance of a single profession at the centre of a framework of care will have shaded into a more fluid system responding variably to patient need.** Clinicians will come together, under different leadership, to manage chronic and episodic conditions. Clinical hierarchies will evolve into affiliations, forming and dissolving according to patient need.

Clinical decisions will be informed by best practice, identified and kept up to date by practitioners and patients working with NICE. Patients will have access to this knowledge as a result of careful dissemination by NICE, using web TV and other electronic media and by working closely with patient advocates. Clinicians will have access through decision support systems on portable and desktop computers, which will also store and collate patient records from a range of sources, inside and outside the health service and which will provide continuous audit data. The clinical guidelines, which will be informed by this knowledge, will be shared across the primary–secondary care interface, securing for patients better integration and appropriate access to hospital based opinion. Essential patient data, together with the electronic key that will allow authorised health service staff to access the full record, will be available to patients to keep with them, in the form of a small card.

Places

The place will be different. When patients need to go to community medical centres, they will be bigger and perhaps more impersonal than even the larger health centres now. Paper will be less in evidence than it is now, replaced increasingly with screens. Many patients will appreciate the speed, efficiency and accuracy of technology. But there will be others who will find it intimidating and will search for the human skills of clinicians. **Remote access to specialists will speed diagnosis and treatment guidelines will allow more care to be provided from primary care medical centres.** Some centres will be big enough to support viable specialist clinics, reducing waiting times, journeys and the time-to-treatment decisions. These larger centres will have patient education areas, which will be used by patients on their own and guided by clinicians. And the more forward thinking clinical groups will be inviting patient groups to join them in their audit meetings and continuing education sessions.

Rewards

Primary care will be an exciting and rewarding place to work. Patients will appreciate the extended role of the clinicians who will be providing their care and the improved environments that the continuous investment in facilities over the next ten years will bring. Care offered in community settings will come of age and will be offered in flexible partnership, rather than in a hierarchy with secondary and tertiary care. It will be consistently good over time and geographically continuously refreshed, with updated knowledge presented in an accessible way. It will be a place where everyone's contribution – patient and clinician – is sought and respected, offering the opportunity for a balanced transaction between patient and carer. It will be a health service to which the people working for the National Institute for Clinical Excellence will have been proud to have contributed.

‹‹‹ Vision 10 ›››

A perspective from a community trust

Lucy Hadfield
Chief Executive, South West London Community NHS Trust
Virtual PCG Board Community Trust Member

BY 2009, THE GOVERNMENT'S RADICAL PROGRAMME TO MODERNISE PRIMARY CARE AND THE NHS should be complete. There will be a universal pattern of respected primary care organisations, providing a range of locally accessible services tailored to meet common health (and perhaps social) needs more effectively than now, and able to arrange for less common needs to be met by fewer hospital providers. If things go well, the country will be even more prosperous and harmonious. Fewer people will suffer and die young from cancer, coronary heart disease and stroke. Medical and technological advances will give more people the chance to avoid ill health. People will be much more confident and proactive about looking after themselves.

In a less rosy picture of 2009, if things do not go quite so well, we might be grappling with a range of problems such as:

› social discord as the gap between the 'haves' and the 'have nots' grows

› increased mental illness in all parts of society as social networks shrink

› difficult ethical choices raised by advances in medical research

› jobs in health care becoming increasingly undervalued, unattractive and unfilled

› unstable health care organisations lurching from one financial crisis to another.

Many factors that will make the difference between these optimistic and pessimistic scenarios are not under the control of those currently responsible for delivery in the NHS. But some factors are. As Chief Executive of a community trust in London in 1999, what should I and my colleagues be doing now and over the next few years to achieve the intended and desired outcomes?

Integrated care

Trends in health care needs are moving towards chronic disease management and health promotion/support to enable people to live healthier lifestyles and prevent disease. Information technology can transform the ways in which health professionals and health systems work to address those needs.

Providing evidence-based care to a patient as part of an integrated pathway, rather than as a series of stand-alone interventions, can be a reality in 2009 with the use of information technology and changes in professional working practices. Details of all health care interventions and transactions can be captured to create the care pathway.

The health record can – and arguably should – be owned by the individual in future, rather than by health professionals or by the state. Aligning the potential of information technology with skills, attitudes and behaviours of health professionals and their organisations for positive outcomes will require skilful leadership and management in my trust and throughout the NHS.

Local partnerships – passing on the baton smoothly

Community services are diverse, often invisible and poorly understood. However, they are an essential part of the foundation for stronger primary care. In the current system, they sit between general practice, social care and acute health care. In the early days of primary care groups (PCGs), with a focus on the needs for change in general practice, leadership of community services must not be neglected. Community services need to change and become more responsive to diversity of need and to patients as consumers. They need to enhance general practice and become an integral part of seamless primary and social care, overcoming current organisational boundary problems.

Community trusts will not be needed in their current form in 2009. However, they are current custodians of hidden primary care 'jewels' such as foot care services and many others. It is important that the jewels are recognised by PCGs, valued and subjected to investment so they can be passed on carefully and smoothly to their new organisational home. Community trusts and their staff are often experts in major service change (such as closing long stay hospitals) and in interagency working. These jewels and competences will be needed by new primary care trusts (PCTs) and must not be lost from the NHS.

Community trusts need to work effectively while in a transitional state over the next few years. They will need to co-lead and support the appropriate pace of change in their local health and social care system, working positively alongside other organisations also in transitional states and maintaining good services to the point of the community trust's transformation or demise. They need to be proactive in their local area, designing the end point, with the other players (that is, when a network of PCTs and possibly other organisations will be robust enough to have replaced many of the current functions of health authorities and community trusts) and the plan to get there. Managing the costs of transition will be a great challenge – smooth handovers require an element of double running costs. It is difficult to see whether and how they will be funded and the risks of financial instability over the next few years are great.

Leadership of an organisation that faces significant downscaling and does not know yet where it is going to end up is particularly challenging. **Mastering the motivation and energy for positive change among the leaders in community trusts needs approaches such as empowerment of staff, loosening of controls and leading from behind rather than the front.**

What about the workers?

There will be dual pressures within primary care both to specialise further to address discrete needs and to integrate a more complex range of resources to address the multiple needs in a larger, more diverse, more knowledgeable and probably more demanding population than the list of the average GP practice of today. These pressures will impact directly on primary care staff and on what they do.

Primary care workers in 2009 will be identifiable – doctors (primarily GPs), dentists, pharmacists, opticians, nurses, therapists and their support staff. The more positive scenarios for 2009 depend on all primary care professionals embracing change themselves. While retaining their distinct and unique contributions to the care pathway that continue to be understood and trusted by the public, health professionals will also need to be more adaptable in applying their expertise, and more knowledgeable and understanding of the contributions of others to the care pathway. They will need enhanced skills in teamwork, use of IT and networking. These will be acquired best through multidisciplinary learning.

More flexibility within community and practice nursing is required. For example, skills associated with health visitors today need to be more widely spread across the primary health care team and school nurses need to refocus on the public health agenda.[1] District nurses will need to develop their assessment and care management functions for complex chronic disease management and also enhance their skills in post-acute and palliative care. Like GPs they will be under pressure both to enhance specialist skills and improve integration skills.

How will health professionals adapt to these pressures? With an increasingly mobile labour market, career pathways need to be more flexible and attractive. The main professional bodies are showing encouraging signs, such as the United Kingdom Central Council for Nursing Midwifery and Health Visiting (UKCCs') recent moves to revise the nursing curriculum to enhance practical learning.[2] There is an urgent need to reform post-registration education systems and the learning environment for all the professions working in primary care if any impact is to be made by 2009.

Primary care will need flexible and innovative organisational frameworks in 2009, both to allow specialists to be self-employed and to attract other staff to be employed in organisations that can assemble and integrate a wider range of different resources for diagnosis, treatment and care. Organisations will need to support continuous and rapid learning.

Organisations employing primary care staff will only succeed if their human resources policies provide the rewards desired by primary care professionals. For staff currently employed by community trusts, these include **family-friendly working schedules and facilities, opportunities for personal and professional development, fair pay, freedom from harassment, discrimination or threats to safety, and opportunities to be involved in decisions that affect their working lives.** Guidance on the establishment of PCTs[3] addresses these requirements. Community services staff would not welcome the possibility of one professional group dominating others.

Health care buildings

The legacy of health care buildings is a barrier to the optimistic scenario. We need to look critically and strategically at the building stock across all health care organisations as today's buildings will not serve us well in 2009. Individual private ownership of many GP practices could be a constraint.

Hospitals and health clinics are tangible evidence of the NHS for the public. **If the benefits of service changes are not clearly understood, health buildings disproportionately symbolise the NHS in the minds of the public and local politicians, and any change is fiercely resisted. We need innovation and investment across all health care players to make the changes to buildings we need and to carry the public with us.**

Keeping the public and ministers informed about progress

During the modernisation of the NHS over the next ten years, it is crucial that channels of communication are fully and equally open amongst ministers, health care managers, health care professionals and the public. We have to manage the change together and listen carefully to each other along the way. We must be guided by and stick to principles of trust, realism, honesty and respect. Our joint goal is better public health, i.e. the optimistic scenario, and the means must be congruent with the end.

References

1. Department of Health. *The New NHS; Modern, Dependable.* 1997.
2. Department of Health. *Making a Difference, Strengthening the nursing, midwifery and health visiting contribution to health and health care.* 1999.
3. HSC 1999/167 Primary Care Trusts: Application Process.

Vision 11

Radical and imaginative initiatives

Lynn Young
Community Health Advisor, Royal College of Nursing
Virtual PCG Board Nurse Member

THE ORIGINAL NHS LEGISLATION WAS BOTH INSPIRATIONAL AND COURAGEOUS. THIS RADICAL action allowed the British public for the first time the luxury of being able to relax over the cost of their health care. However, it has also been acknowledged that since the early days of the NHS, primary health care has struggled to achieve a significant level of power and influence. Even before 1950 it became abundantly clear which parts of the NHS were calling the tune and receiving the lion's share of available resources. The secondary sector – hospitals, especially the teaching variety – became far too powerful and consumed (and still do) almost 75 per cent of the NHS fund.

Fifty plus years later, as we face a new century, a number of health enthusiasts struggle to consider how a modern and effective health service can be developed within the inevitable cost constraints. **But radical and imaginative initiatives have already started to happen and it feels as if primary health care has truly arrived.**

1999

Current health and social policies focus on setting up systems which, given time, will change behaviour and attitudes and put primary health care in the driving seat of the NHS. As we approach the end of the 20th century it feels as if it is a great time to be a primary health care groupie!

While chaos, turbulence, frenetic energy and confusion flourish, an enormous level of commitment also prevails in the world of community health to ensure that the NHS becomes truly modernised. The timescale set by the Government means that much change has to happen in a short space of time. The present upheaval within the NHS and local government means that it is essential for us to keep a close eye on the plot and maintain a realistic vision of what we wish to achieve in the future.

So, given the Government's health modernisation agenda what can we expect primary health care to look like by the year 2005?

> will the public notice any difference?

> will bright young things want to work and remain working in the new NHS?

> will health care services provide a significant level of evidence-based practice and be more effective?

> is it realistic to hope for a reduction in the present unacceptable health inequalities and improved public health for the citizens of our most impoverished communities?

Well informed optimists working in the NHS believe that the current health and social policies are right and that primary health care workers have a new and huge opportunity to help improve the nation's health.

2005

Primary care groups (PCGs) have been recognised as a learning exercise and have disappeared into the sunset, along with fundholding and the internal market. A grand national event is being planned by the NHS Executive to celebrate the good news that by the start of 2006 the whole of the British public will receive personalised community health services from their local primary care trust. Hospital staff now understand and welcome the shift in power and control, believing this change to be in the best interest of the people they care for. **The drive to carry out treatments in accordance with clinical pathways, guidelines and protocols has resulted in improved continuity of care and better outcomes in terms of health gain for patients.** Furthermore, strong partnerships between hospital and community clinicians have developed since the late 1990s, which has helped the NHS – and primary health care in particular – to be in great condition!

Independent, self-employed GPs still flourish, but in the 21st century a growing number of salaried GPs have welcomed the opportunity to be employed by primary care trusts (PCTs). This is not surprising, as PCTs have developed into successful, family friendly and enlightened organisations that offer attractive employment conditions and professional development opportunities to their staff. Newly qualified doctors, nurses and therapists experience great competition to enjoy working in the 'engine' of the NHS – primary health care.

Nursing continues to develop in leaps and bounds. Nurse managed NHS Direct, walk-in centres and healthy living centres have certainly made an impact on traditional NHS structures. Nurses are now the new and more appropriate gateway to the NHS, rather than GPs. The drive to persuade the public to improve their health, take greater personal responsibility and be more independent has been achieved. Publicity campaigns, modern nursing practice and greater multidisciplinary co-operation have contributed towards this success.

Clinicians have confronted their personal practice and worked alongside people to help them self-care and be more responsible for their own health. Simple health problems are mostly dealt with by individuals, who no longer feel the need to consult doctors and nurses. People feel reassured that they can access nurses and doctors when they want to and this has encouraged more, not less, self-care. Most importantly, trivial health problems that can be self-managed no longer place unnecessary demands on primary health care services. People are certainly better informed and confident about looking after themselves, their friends and families. The healthy lifestyle message has at last been heard and inwardly digested by a vast section of the public.

Children have received so much relevant health education via the national curriculum that the nation has high hopes for the health of the next adult generation.

Primary care trusts are responsible for making the major decisions on how public money is spent on local health services. Difficult rationing decisions are made closely with members of the local community and there are great efforts to ensure that the public is kept well informed when a service ceases to be provided or new ones are introduced. Systems of clinical governance ensure that standards of care are for the main part exemplary and all clinicians make great efforts to keep their practice up to date and in accordance with the most recent evidence and research.

Widespread models of multidisciplinary peer review, clinical supervision and shared learning initiatives have helped to develop a great number of well supported integrated primary health care team (PHCT) members whose morale and level of job satisfaction are high.

One interesting effect of the new and modern NHS is the fact that the public no longer believe that the local hospital is the answer to their health problems. Hospital beds are only used for people during critical incidents. Even intensive nursing and therapies are provided within the sanctity of peoples' homes.

Conclusion

Primary health care workers who are presently (1999) working hard to make sense of Mr Blair's reforms should be confident that their efforts to develop modern health will be successful. During this time of great change and new developments we need to believe that successful primary health care can contribute to that great and inspirational ideal – reduced health inequalities and improved public health by the year 2005.

Nurse-led primary care

Sue Baker
Health Visitor, South West London Community NHS Trust
Virtual PCG Board Nurse Member

PRIMARY CARE GROUPS (PCGS) HAVE INTRODUCED A RADICAL CHANGE TO THE WAY primary care is provided. This development has created new opportunities for nurses and will have a profound effect on the way primary care is provided by 2009. Devolving commissioning down from health authorities to PCGs has fostered a pluralist approach to primary care, an approach that requires joint governance and corporate action. Nurses have found themselves with an opportunity to extend their roles in the leadership and strategic development of primary care services.

The contribution of community nurses in Health Improvement Programmes has been, and will continue to be, influential in shaping services according to need. Nurse-led personal medical services pilots have heralded the way for nurse-led services by 2009. Nurses have proved capable of delivering primary care, buying in sessions or directly employing GPs. Increasingly, nurses, who offer a personal and cost effective service, can manage patients suffering from minor self-limiting illnesses or stable chronic diseases. Benchmarking these pilots and comparison with equivalent service providers will enable the service to improve continually through actions resulting from the setting of targets and monitoring of outcomes. Electronic health records, access to the national electronic library for health and **electronic access to national/local protocols and standards of care will be essential if multiprofessional services are to work effectively.**

Nurse-led primary care should not be seen to compete with general practice, but complement it in areas where there is a large amount of unmet need, such as providing a first port of call to assess the health needs of immigrants and homeless people. By using a variety of professional groups, nurse-led centres will be able to manage a wide spectrum of needs under one roof, from dealing with minor ailments to family planning, childcare, mental health care and midwifery services.

Unfortunately the recruitment and retention of nurses is not likely to improve dramatically over the next decade as other career opportunities compete for an ever-dwindling number of eligible recruits. Managing skill mix in nursing teams will become increasingly important to run the service well. **Nurses will need to become more innovative in the ways they work. This is already taking place in integrated nursing teams where members of the primary care nursing teams pool their resources to benefit patient/client care.** Breaking down professional tribalism is essential if problems of recruitment are to be addressed. This will be helped by establishing a central core curriculum for all community nurse training, including practice nursing, and by giving nurses the opportunity to become multi-qualified, maximising their skills and knowledge in different fields of community nursing.

The opportunities for nurses to diversify are enormous. For instance, health visitors are trained in public health nursing, yet the majority find themselves focusing on the care of families with children under five.

Innovation involves an element of risk taking and uncertainty. Erosion of professional boundaries may lead to greater uncertainty and lower morale. For nurses to take over some of the traditional tasks currently carried out by GPs requires the legal infrastructure to be reviewed. The regulations for nurse prescribing only allow those community nurses holding a health visiting or district nurse qualification to prescribe independently from a very limited formulary. This will hinder the progress of nurse-led centres.

Professional roles need to become clearly defined if new areas of work are to be exploited. In addition, the area of risk management, personal liability and professional negligence will need careful consideration. Nurses will require training and support to feel confident in any new role.[1]

If future policy makers address these concerns, they will enable nurses to achieve greater autonomy. Primary care nurses so empowered will be able to use their knowledge and skills to improve a wide range of health care services for patients in 2009.

References
1. Williams A, Sibbald B. *Journal of Advanced Nursing* 1999; 29 (3): 737–45.

‹‹‹ Vision 13 ›››

The ideal primary care service

Donna Covey
Director, Association of Community Health Councils of England and Wales
Virtual PCG Board Lay Member

THE HEALTH SERVICE BELONGS TO US ALL. WE PAY FOR IT THROUGH OUR TAXES, AND WE USE IT throughout our lives. Primary care reform will have worked if, in ten years time, ordinary people once again feel an ownership of the health service.

Imagine a Patient-centred primary care service in 2009. When you book your appointment, you are treated as a valued service user. **It is possible to get an appointment that fits in with the rest of your life and does not mean taking a whole morning off work, or arranging for someone else to pick the children up from school.** There will be central guidelines across the country about how long you have to wait to see a GP or other primary care health care provider. These guidelines will be adhered to, wherever you live. And you can call to make the appointment at any time. No longer do you have to ring every five minutes during the window of opportunity when the surgery phone is being answered, in the hope that you will eventually get through. No longer will you have to force yourself to stay awake when you are ill and need to sleep, because you are worried that you will not wake up in time to ring the surgery before their phone switches back into answer machine mode. And no more waiting, frightened and in pain, to be able to make the call to make the appointment that will give you peace of mind.

You can send an e-mail, go to sleep, and when you wake up your mail will include an appointment date and time.

And when you get to the primary care centre, walking in the door will not automatically make you feel worse. The local health centre is a warm and welcoming place. Not painted institutional green or rented flat magnolia (guaranteed to make you feel ill when all you have come for is a routine smear test). The notice boards tell you what the services are and how to access them. The poster telling you how to make a complaint is bigger than A4, and can be read without a magnifying glass. The poster next to it telling you how to feed in your views on how the service could be changed and improved is even bigger and brighter.

There is a system that allows you to use the toilet without missing your appointment. If you have a long wait, there is somewhere to get coffee, tea and mineral water. There are toys for children to play with as well as magazines for the adults. The local communities know how to donate books, magazines and toys to the local health centre, and so there are plenty to go round, and they are in good condition.

It is a one-stop shop. Doctors, practice nurses, physiotherapists, chiropractors, dieticians and other service providers all have space in the centre, at different points in the week.

If your appointment is a referral from your GP for another practice based service, then it will be checked with you – before you receive it. You no longer have to make three phone calls – one to explain you cannot do next Wednesday, another to confirm you would like another appointment, and a third to explain that no, you cannot do tomorrow at such short notice, and why do they use second class post rather than a telephone or the e-mail? You may even be able to arrange the appointment at the time the doctor suggests a referral – after all, you will be in the building.

If you need to be referred on from primary care, you will be kept informed. No long, silent waits thinking you have been forgotten. No day-before cancellations. And, above all, information. You will be told when you can expect to hear. If there is a delay, you will be told why.

The ethos of the service will be different. It will be a local service that is owned by, and responsive to, the local community. A local service that offers patients informed choices, treats them as intelligent adults and involves them in strategic as well as individual decision-making.

In my 2009, patients are the experts. Not just in the needs of our own condition, but in the strategic needs of our local communities as well. And we are experts not just when we are sick, but also when we are well. After all, that's when we feel most able to put time and energy into making suggestions about improvements.

The local paper keeps us updated on issues facing the local primary care services. It tells us what is new, what is changing and how our voices can be heard.

The local community health council (CHC) has a decent budget in 2009, when we have finally realised that greater public involvement makes the health service better. They are running regular discussion groups in the area. Funding provides for an outreach worker, so that hard-to-reach groups get their voice heard too, even if they cannot get to meetings. All patients now have a right to be supported by the CHC in a complaint, and the funding provides for specialist staff to do this. Information from the CHC's listening activities, and suggestions for improvements thrown up by their complaints work, are fed into the regular meetings of the primary care trust board. The CHC has speaking rights at meetings, and can place items on the agenda. They are listened to with respect, because the service recognises it is the voice of the public that must be heard, not just that of the professionals and the local worthies. And the board itself is diverse, reflecting the local population.

And the best thing of all about my vision of 2009 is that it can be done without another Act of Parliament. Patient-centred primary care is about changing attitudes. It could happen.

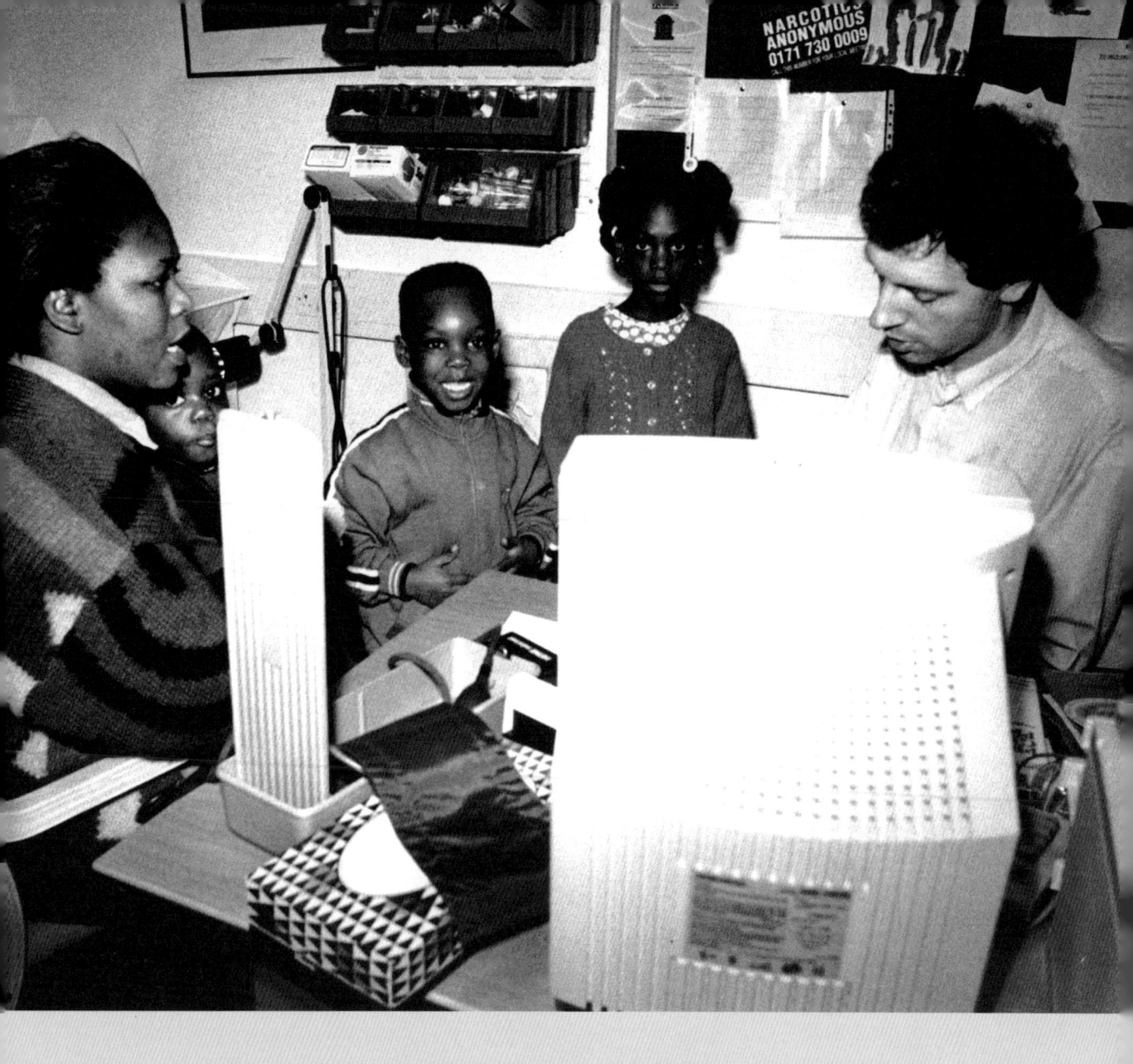

It is possible to get an appointment that fits in with the rest of your life and does not mean taking a whole morning off work, or arranging for someone else to pick the children up from school.

Lambeth in 2009

Judith Brodie
*Secretary for Social Services and Health Improvement,
London Borough of Lambeth
Virtual PCG Board Social Services Member*

THINKING BACK TO 1999 I CAN REMEMBER A TIME OF HIGH ASPIRATIONS BUT SERVICE AND organisational flux. At the time I was responsible for social services and health in Lambeth, one of the most deprived boroughs in the country. It is hard to believe now, but at that time memories were still fresh of the corruption and chaos that had characterised the borough in the 1980s and early 1990s, and were still affecting its ability to change and become the beacon borough now familiar to us. Health was new on the borough's corporate agenda although joint work with social services was established. Primary care groups (collectives of GP practices) had just been launched and were finding their feet.

Looking back, we can see that the seeds of a different system had been sown, but the shoots were not even peering over the soil.

Communities

I have just received through my door the 2009 community plan. It is fascinating to flick through it and see what has been happening.

> ❯ St Margaret's Neighbourhood has a high number of families but **teenage pregnancies have plummeted since a task force of young people decided they wanted to do something about it.** They consulted widely and found many young people did not like going to doctors and did not take lessons on sexual health seriously. We now have community health workers who combine nursing advice and information on sexual health and other issues with youth work focusing on healthy lifestyles. A stronger

education system that has increased the educational attainment and the aspirations and confidence of many young women has also contributed.

> There is a new borough director of health, who has come from one of the healthy living centres. Kennwell Healthy Living was radical when it was set up, in having a very small central base, with most staff working out in the neighbourhoods – in community centres, community schools and town centres. The healthy living centre started as a local volunteer project linking healthy community work with work experience and training and development opportunities. It has evolved into a major health promotion resource for local people, rooted firmly in the community.

> Another Living Well centre has just opened in a neighbourhood high street. It offers medical diagnoses and advice and is fully equipped, with telemedicine links to the local specialist clinicians. People can have their annual health audit there. They receive their healthy living prescription and are immediately helped to fill it – for example, with exercise sessions, stress buster workshops or smokestop programmes. One of the big success stories has been the extent to which many employers have been involved. Unfortunately, despite the European Healthy Working Directive, many employers still do only the minimum to promote a healthy workplace.

> Part of the Living Well Centre is a healthy living library with consumer information on health promotion and on a wide range of conditions, in paper and virtual form. This includes information about local sports and leisure activities, health awareness workshops and food co-ops. There is instant video access to LanguageLink interpreters for minority communities and people with hearing impairment and all material can immediately be taped or produced in large print for people with visual impairment. There is also an optician in the centre.

Progress

Technology has transformed the way we do things. The Internet and video links are now available in every household, thanks to digital TV in the early 2000s and the government's Information Equity Strategy. This means users and the public can regularly be consulted about borough or neighbourhood priorities or specific service development issues. Responses have been patchy, so the government is proposing a legal requirement for people to respond to the annual citizens' survey (as well as the census) if sampled, and only to be able to evade Citizens Jury Service for a very good reason.

The transfer of health commissioning to local authorities was a significant step in enabling faster progress. Many GPs were not supportive but, by then, whole borough primary care trusts had been commissioning for a couple of years and it began to make sense to bring their responsibilities under one common public service umbrella, and bring democratic accountability to the health service. While the cultural differences made this a difficult transition, it certainly made it easier to develop some of the new services. Community carers now deliver health and care at home, and five health care centres now commission and deliver many community health and social care services. Housing and benefits advice and information are also available there. Mental health services are delivered by the national Mental Health Agency.

GP consultations are fundamentally the same. While there are many more nurse specialists, many people still visit their GP. However, a high proportion have first called NHS Direct and made the appointment through them, having first sought advice from an NHS Direct nurse.

Information on the approved drugs list is widely available and the screens in every pharmacy help patients to find out information about various medications. While this has helped to clarify the debate about rationing, many people remember drugs that are not now available on the NHS or find out about treatments available in other countries through the Internet. As a result, private GPs have done a roaring trade.

Conclusion

Ten years is not such a long time in the scheme of things, although some major changes have taken place. One thing has not changed. Public services are still changing. Service and organisational flux are a way of life.

Community pharmacy 2009: would you believe it?

Colin Baldwin
Pharmacy Development Controller, Boots
Virtual PCG Board co-opted Community Pharmacist

YOU MAY FIND IT HARD TO BELIEVE – BUT WE COMMUNITY PHARMACISTS DIDN'T ALWAYS HAVE such an important role in primary care as we do now. Ten years ago in 1999 – back in the last century – we used few of the skills which are now taken for granted by patients and those who looked to us for help, advice and support in staying fit, healthy and well. True – we did play an important part in supplying medicines on prescription and helping patients to treat minor ailments – but we were somehow not a part of primary care and public health in the way that we are now.

Thinking back it was the creation of primary care groups and the re-engineering of primary and social care that provided the opportunity for community pharmacists to become partners in the planning and delivery of health care for the community. Until then it had not been appreciated that community pharmacists were not just experts in medicines, but also had the natural ability to work with patients and their GPs to ensure that maximum benefit was obtained from medicines. **In those days nobody would have imagined the way in which pharmacists now manage the medication for a PCG's patients. Nobody could have imagined the savings in drug costs, reductions in secondary care referrals and the improvements in outcomes which are now commonplace.**

Nobody realised either at that time that community pharmacists had important strategic, business and planning skills to bring to the development of primary care provision. We all now take for granted the contribution of the community pharmacists on the primary care trust executives, but their unique insight into patients and their local communities hasn't always been used in the development of local primary care planning. Amazing, isn't it!

Do you know, back in those days, while there were 15,000 pharmacies, readily accessible to the vast majority of people – with the constant availability of a pharmacist over long hours – these pharmacies had no computer links with GPs or other members of the primary care team. Incredible! There was no formal way in which the community pharmacist could advise a patient's doctor of interventions undertaken in the pharmacy – no way of formally alerting the doctor of problems with compliance or therapeutic efficacy. Of course, all that has changed now – no longer is there a period of 'radio silence' for the GP after the patient has left the surgery with their prescription. The community pharmacist is now part of the team receiving and transmitting information. Some of you may even remember that prescriptions were actually printed on pieces of paper that patients took to the pharmacy for dispensing, even though smart cards, store cards and cashless transactions were commonplace.

I can hardly believe this myself – but ten years ago community pharmacists made very little contribution to health promotion and health education. True, most pharmacies had displays of health promotion leaflets and many took part in co-ordinated campaigns on important subjects such as smoking cessation and skin cancer. Some community pharmacists even ran health education clinics – but nobody it seems had realised how effective pharmacists could be in influencing their customers' and patients' behaviours. In particular, it hadn't been appreciated that pharmacists were not only respected by the public for their knowledge of medicines but they were approachable and able to discuss treatments and inform patients in an interesting, understandable and engaging way. In these days of the World Wide Web, when there is no shortage of information, the pharmacist is relied upon to interpret and tailor it for individuals. I remember, back in the last century it being recognised that community pharmacists had daily access to most of the women in the population as customers and through them to their families. It took the formation of PCGs and the focus on local planning of primary care delivery to realise the value of such access in terms of health promotion and health education.

Ten years ago community pharmacists didn't prescribe for NHS patients as they do now. Patients had to go to their GP for treatment of minor illness and there were no arrangements for repeat prescribing by pharmacists for chronic conditions. It is perhaps not surprising that GPs had such difficulty in coping with their workload and the demand on A&E services became heavier and heavier.

NHS Direct and walk-in centres undoubtedly played their part and continue to do so in releasing GPs' time to focus on priorities. But who could have foreseen the key role which community pharmacy has played in the setting up of NHS walk-in centres in easily acceptable retail locations, and the role which pharmacists play in both providing immediate advice alongside nurses on the NHS Direct lines and also in being available to provide services to NHS Direct patients referred to them.

Ten years ago there was little appreciation of the enormous private investment that supported the community pharmacy service and infrastructure. Curiously, it was only when PCTs were formed and opportunities created to consider alternative mechanisms for supplying pharmaceutical services that the true value of the community pharmacy network came to be realised. Here was a living and highly efficient example of public–private partnership, which then and today works to the benefit of patients, the NHS and health professionals.

Finally, let me remind you of those services pharmacists provide now that they didn't just a few years ago in 1999:

> medication management and support services, working with GPs and patients to optimise the effectiveness of treatment

> prescribing for minor illnesses and chronic conditions

> health promotion and health education as an integral partner in the local health agenda

> strategic planning at primary care team executive level where their business skills are much valued

> provision of space for walk-in centres and clinics

> an important participating role in NHS Direct.

References
1. Department of Health. *Saving Lives, Our Healthier Nation*. 1999.
2. Department of Health. *The New NHS; Modern, Dependable*. 1997.